ENGLISH FOR NURSES

David Austin
and
Tim Crosfield

Longman

LONGMAN GROUP UK LIMITED
Longman House, Burnt Mill, Harlow,
Essex CM20 2JE, England
and Associated Companies throughout the world.

First published by Hermods under the title
of English in Hospital 1 and 2

This edition first published by
Longman Group Limited in one volume
in association with Hermods and
Tjänstemänens Bildningsverksamhet

Twenty-first impression 1994

Produced through Longman Malaysia, VVP

ISBN 0 – 582 – 55019 – X

Contents

1 — Where Do You Work?

Nurse Smith	Where do you work?
Nurse Robinson	I work at Saint Peter's, in a surgical ward. And you – where do you work?
Nurse Smith	I work in an orthopaedic ward at Queen Mary's. I'm an S.R.N. Are you an S.R.N?
Nurse Robinson	No, I'm not. I'm a student nurse.

And where do you work?

I work in ....

at ....

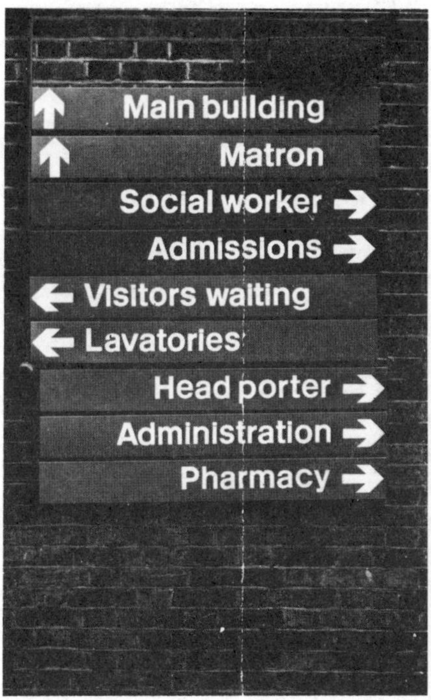

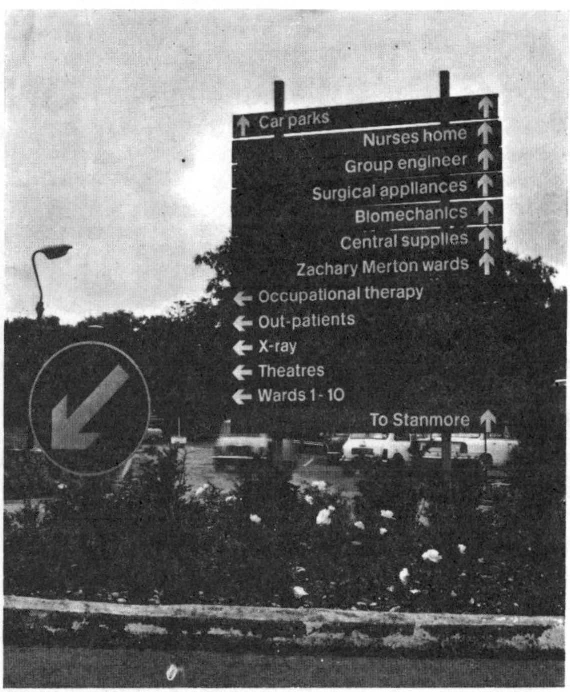

A

Some Wards and Departments

Surgical Ward ....

Medical Ward ....

Orthopaedic Ward ....

Gynaecological Ward ....

Geriatric Ward ....

Paediatric Ward ....

Dermatological Ward ....

E.N.T. Ward ....

Long-stay Ward ....

Intensive Care Unit ....

X-ray Department ....

Operating Theatre ....

Casualty and Emergency Department (or Unit) (or Accident and Emergency Department) ....

....

Central Sterile Supply Department ....

....

Dispensary ....

Laboratory ....

Out-Patients' Clinic ....

Maternity Unit ....

Occupational Therapy Department ....

....

Physiotherapy Department ....

....

Antenatal Clinic ....

Post-Natal Clinic ....

Psychiatric Unit ....

Admissions Department ....

Infectious Diseases Unit ....

Anaesthetic Room ....

B

What do they do?

radiolog*ist*	radiolog*y*	radiolog*ical*
psychologist	psychology	psychological
dermatologist	dermatology	dermatological
gynaecologist	gynaecology	gynaecological
venerologist	venerology	venerological
pathologist	pathology	pathological
histologist	histology	histological
cytologist	cytology	cytological
haematologist	haematology	haematological
bacteriologist	bacteriology	bacteriological
obstetric*ian*	obstetric*s*	obstetric (*al*)
paediatrician	paediatrics	paediatric
geriatrician	geriatrics	geriatric
psychiatr*ist*	psychiatr*y*	psychiatr*ic*
anaesthetist	anaesthetics	anaesthetic
surgeon	surgery	surgical
physician	medicine	medical
orthopaedic surgeon	orthopaedics	orthopaedic

C

Who does what?

Someone who studies and practises dermatology is a *dermatologist*.
Someone who studies and practises radiology is a *radiologist*.

Someone who studies and practises

1 gynaecology is a ....

2 bacteriology is a ....

3 histology is a ....

4 venerology is a ....

5 psychology is a ....

6 pathology is a ....

D

Where could you find

1 a dermatologist? In a .... ward.

2 a radiologist? In an .... department.

3 an obstetrician? In a .... unit.

4 a surgeon? In an .... theatre.

5 a physician? In a .... ward.

6 a paediatrician? In a .... ward.

E

Someone who studies

1 .... is an orthopaedic surgeon.

2 blood is a ....

3 the body's cells is a ....

4 .... is a gynaecologist.

5 anaesthetics is an ....

6 .... is a surgeon.

2 — Parts of the Body

Male–anterior aspect

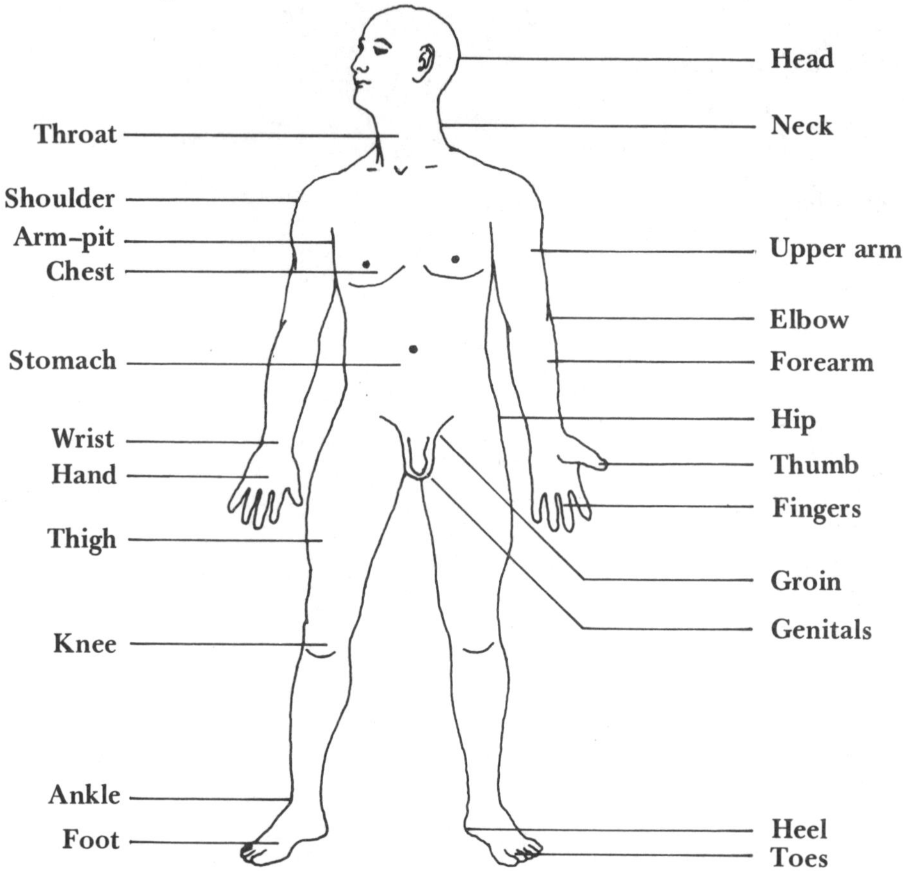

A

Aches and pains

A pain	A swelling	Sprained	To ache
An ache	A graze	Stiff	To hurt
A bruise	A sting	Sore	To throb
A rash	A bite		To itch
A cut			To irritate
A scar			

I have (I've got) a pain in my chest.
My chest hurts.
My chest aches.

He has (he's got) a pain in his stomach.
His stomach hurts.
His stomach aches.

You have (you've got) a pain in your elbow.
Your elbow hurts.
Your elbow aches.

She has (she's got) a pain in her leg.
Her leg hurts.
Her leg aches.

Female – anterior aspect

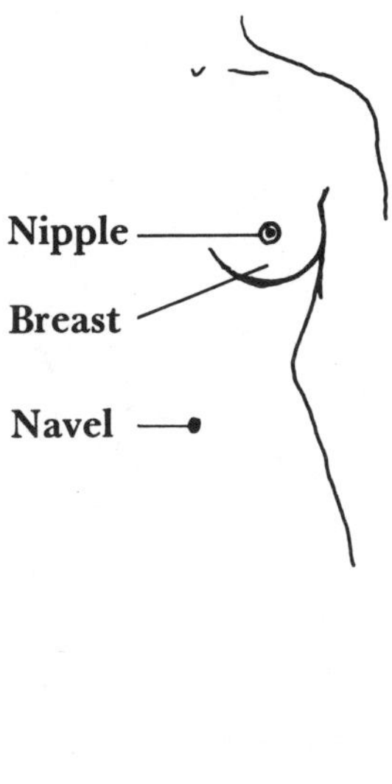

Male – posterior aspect

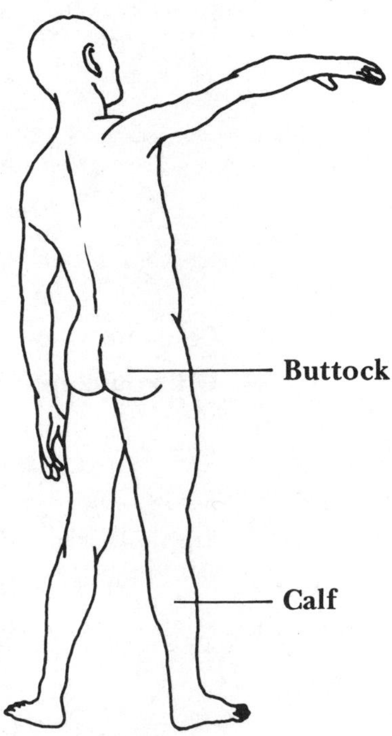

Drills: Polite requests

Come in!

Come in, please!

Will you come in/, please/?

Would you come in/, please/?

Would you mind standing up/, please/?

Patients in hospital are usually anxious and fearful. It is important that hospital staff put them at their ease, by being polite and pleasant. The following drills teach you polite forms in English. Be careful about the way your voice rises and falls when you say these sentences. Listen to the way the teacher says the sentences.

Drill 1

Command	Come in.
Request	Come in, please!

Change these commands to polite requests. Be careful to make your voice rise and fall correctly

1 Come in.
2 Sit down.
3 Stand up.
4 Turn round.
5 Say Ah.
6 Turn over.
7 Bend down.
8 Lie down.
9 Sit up.
10 Look up.

Drill 2

Command	Come in.
Request	Will you come in, please?

1 Raise your arm
2 Move your head.
3 Lift your leg.
4 Arch your back.
5 Lower your foot.
6 Open your mouth.
7 Put out your tongue.
8 Bend your knees.
9 Touch your toes.
10 Wriggle your fingers.

Drill 3

Command	Come in.
Request	Would you come in, please?

1 Roll your sleeve up.
2 Take your shirt off.
3 Hold your head up.
4 Hold your breath in.
5 Take your trousers off.
6 Keep your mouth open.
7 Keep your eyes shut.
8 Go to C.S.S.D.

Drill 4

Command	Stand up.
Request	Would you mind standing up, please?

1 Stand up.
2 Sit down.
3 Lie down.
4 Turn over.
5 Sit up.
6 Turn round.
7 Bend down.
8 Roll your sleeve up.

B

Where is the pain?

Look at the figure and complete the following sentences.

He has a pain in his 1 ....

He has a stiff 2 ....

He has a sting on his 3 ....

He has a rash on his 4 ....

He has a graze on his 5 ....

He has a pain in his 6 ....

He has a cut on his 7 ....

His 8 .... hurts.

He has a scar on his 9 ....

His 10 .... aches.

He has a sprained 11 ....

He has a sore 12 ....

He has a bruise on his 13 ....

He has a swelling on his 14 ....

He has a pain in his 15 ....

He has cuts on his 16 ....

He has a swelling in his 17 ....

His 18 .... ache.

He has a pain in his 19 ....

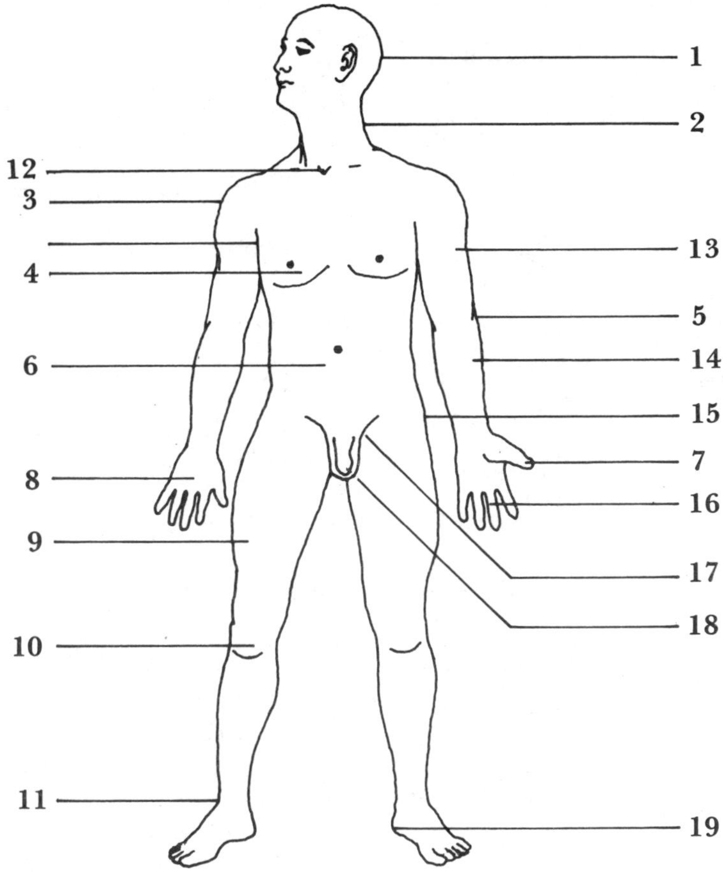

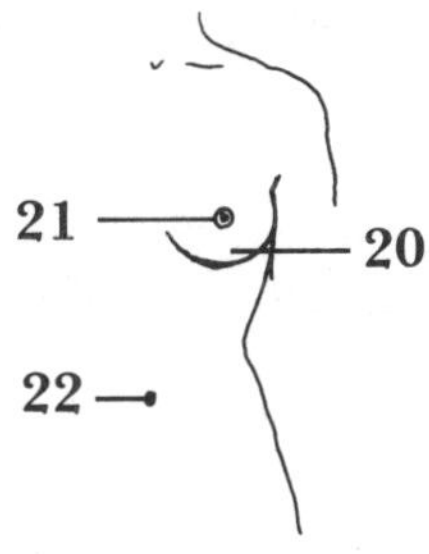

She has a sore 20 . . . .

She has a pain in her 21 . . . .

She has a rash in her 22 . . . .

C

Put in the correct word from this list

off, to, back, in, on, down, by, up, through, round, near

1 Ask the patient to come .... and sit ....

2 Ask the patient to stand .... and turn ....

3 Will you lie .... on the couch, please?

4 Would you roll .... your sleeve?

5 Ask Mr Smith to take .... his coat.

6 Bend .... and touch your toes, please.

7 Take .... your trousers, please.

8 Ask the patient to turn his head .... the left.

9 Will you put .... your clothes, please?

10 Come .... next week, please.

D

Complete the following sentences with the correct word from this list

your, his, her, my, our, its, their

1 Tell Mrs Smith to raise .... right arm.

2 Would you straighten .... left leg, please?

3 The baby has a pain in .... stomach.

4 John has a cut on .... thigh.

5 Ask me to lower .... arm.

6 You have a rash on .... shoulders.

7 He's got a scar on .... left forearm.

3 — Jane Johnson

Jane Johnson works in a surgical ward in a London hospital. Jane does shift work, so she does not go to work at the same time every day. When she is on an early shift, she goes on duty at 7 a.m. and comes off duty at 3 p.m. Late shifts start at 2 p.m. and finish at 10 p.m. Jane does not like late shifts.

Jane always goes to work by bus when she is on an early shift. The bus stops outside the out-patients' department. When she is on a late shift, Jane generally walks from her home to the hospital. When she comes off duty at 10 p.m., she is usually rather tired, and takes the bus home. Sometimes she goes to the taxi-rank outside the main entrance of the hospital and goes home by taxi.

Jane is not a qualified nurse. She is a student nurse, so she does not work in the ward every day. On certain days, she has to attend lectures on general nursing, anatomy and physiology, hygiene and various other subjects. She wants to pass the State Final examinations and become a State Registered Nurse. As a State Registered Nurse she becomes a staff nurse and can, in time, become a sister or even a nursing officer.

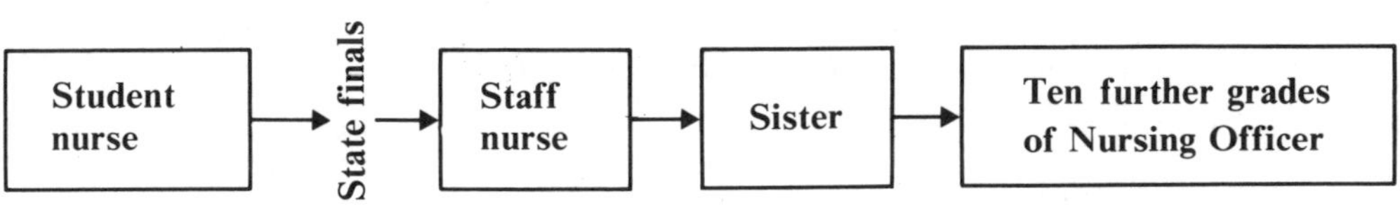

A

Answer the following questions

1 Where does Jane Johnson work?

2 At what time does she go on duty when she is on an early shift?

3 When does she come off duty when she is on an early shift?

4 At what time do late shifts start?

5 When do late shifts finish?

6 When does Jane go to work by bus?
7 Where does the bus stop?
8 When does Jane walk from her home to the hospital?
9 When does she take the bus home?
10 What lectures does Jane attend?
11 What can she become when she has passed the State Final examinations?

B

Read through the second paragraph of the text and underline all the words that can answer the question 'How often'?

Negatives with do and does: Look at these sentences

Jane *works* in a medical ward.	Jane *doesn't work* in a medical ward.
He *always goes* home by taxi.	He *doesn't always go* home by taxi.
It *stops* outside the main gate.	It *doesn't stop* outside the main gate.
I *go* to work at 7 o'clock.	I *don't go* to work at 7 o'clock.
We *always take* the bus home.	We *don't always take* the bus home.
They *finish* work at 6.30 p.m.	They *don't finish* work at 6.30 p.m.

C

Put the following sentences into the negative

1 She works in the x-ray department.
2 He usually studies hard.
3 She often walks past the operating theatre.
4 We have to stay until 10 o'clock.
5 I want to attend lectures.
6 It stops outside the hospital.
7 She does shift work.
8 You finish at 12 o'clock.

Questions with do and does: Look at these sentences

You *do* shift work.	*Do* you *do* shift work?
We *go* on duty at 3 p.m.	*Do* we *go* on duty at 3 p.m.?

I *pass* the surgical ward.	*Do* I *pass* the surgical ward?
They generally *finish* late.	*Do* they generally *finish* late?
She *wants* to go home now.	*Does* she *want* to go home now?
He usually *does* a late shift.	*Does* he usually *do* a late shift?
It *stops* near the hospital.	*Does* it *stop* near the hospital?

D

Make questions from these sentences

1 Jane works in a surgical ward.
2 She does shift work.
3 They go on duty at 2 p.m.
4 The late shift finishes at 10 p.m.
5 We walk past the out-patients' department.
6 She studies hard.
7 The nurse generally walks to work.
8 The bus stops outside the main gate.
9 You have to attend lectures.
10 He usually finishes at 12 o'clock.

Drill 1 I, she, he and it

I work in a hospital. – And Jane? *She works in a hospital, too.*
I do shift work. – And Mr Brown? *He does shift work, too.*

I work in a surgical ward. – And Mary?
I go to work by bus. – And John?
I come off duty at 7.30 p.m. – And Jane?
I walk past the operating theatre. – And the staff nurse?
I often help the sister. – And Jane?
I start at 7 a.m. – And the early shift?
I usually finish at 12 o'clock. – And Jane?
I always study hard. – And Peter?
I attend lectures every day. – And John?
I want to pass the State Finals. – And Jane?
I have to go home now. – And Mary?
I work in the x-ray department. – And Sister Smith?

Drill 2 Questions with do and does

Ask if Jane works in a surgical ward.	*Does Jane work in a surgical ward?*
Ask if buses stop outside the gate.	*Do buses stop outside the gate?*

Ask if Jane goes on duty at 7 a.m.
Ask if they come off duty at 3 p.m.
Ask if the patients often help the staff nurse.
Ask if she usually does split shifts.
Ask if he always goes to work by bus.
Ask if buses stop outside the hospital.
Ask if Jane works in the out-patients' department.
Ask if the nurses attend lectures.

Drill 3 Ask the patient

Ask the patient about his eyes.	*Do your eyes hurt?*
Ask the patient about his head.	*Does your head hurt?*

Ask the patient about his

1	back	4	left arm	7	stomach	10	fingers
2	foot	5	right thigh	8	toes		
3	ears	6	heels	9	chest		

Drill 4 Answer these questions

Do your ears ache?	No.	*No, they don't.*
Do your elbows hurt?	Yes.	*Yes, they do.*
Does your stomach ache?	Yes.	*Yes, it does.*

1	Does your chest hurt?	Yes.
2	Does your back ache?	No.
3	Do your ears hurt?	No.
4	Does your leg ache?	Yes.
5	Do your eyes ache?	No.
6	Does it hurt here?	Yes.
7	Does it hurt there?	No.
8	Do your shoulders ache?	Yes.

4 — Jane on the Wards

Do you remember Jane Johnson? She and her friend Joan Chapman are both nurses. They work at Saint Peter's Hospital, a large teaching hospital in London. Joan did her training at St. Peter's and last year she passed her State Finals and qualified. She is an S.R.N. She is now working as a staff nurse in a men's medical ward.

Jane is a student nurse and is still training. Last month she worked in one of the hospital's surgical wards. She learned to set trolleys for sterile procedures such as surgical dressings, intravenous infusion and catheterization. She carried out certain procedures herself and assisted doctors with others. She often had to go to the central sterile supply department to fetch sterile dressing packs. Sometimes she took patients to the x-ray department or to the occupational therapy unit.

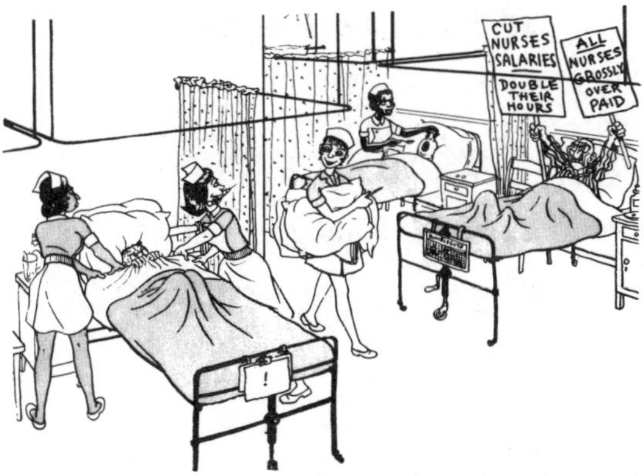

'He's a bit niggly because I confiscated a bottle of Scotch he'd smuggled under the sheets"

London Express Service.

This month Jane is working in the same ward as Joan. She is learning to nurse patients suffering from diseases such as cardiac infarction, cerebral haemorrhage, cerebral thrombosis and pneumonia. At the moment, she is helping a staff nurse to give injections. The staff nurse is explaining to her the doses, action and side effects of the drugs they are administering.

The other nurses in the ward are carrying out various nursing duties. Some are doing bed-baths, one is helping a patient to get out of bed, and another is taking t.p.rs. A doctor is doing a ward round and a physiotherapist is helping a pneumonia-patient to do deep-breathing exercises.

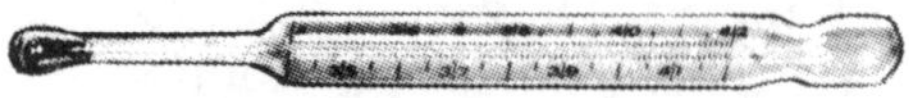

rectal thermometer

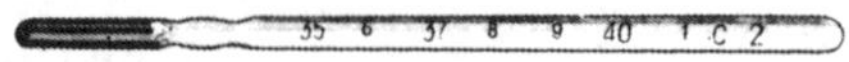

clinical thermometer

A

Answer these questions

1 What sort of hospital is St. Peter's?
2 Where did Joan do her training?
3 When did Joan pass her State Finals?
4 Which ward is Joan working in now?
5 Where did Jane work last month?
6 Which sterile procedures did she learn to set trolleys for?
7 Where did she go to fetch sterile dressing packs?
8 Where did she sometimes take patients?
9 Where is Jane working this month?
10 Which patients is Jane learning to nurse?
11 What is she doing at the moment?
12 What is the staff nurse explaining to her?

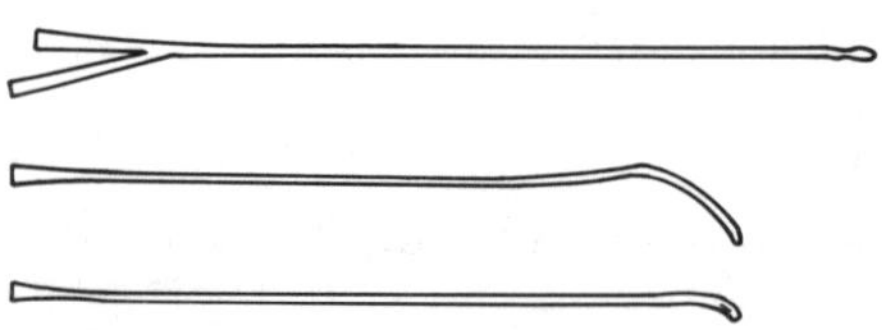

catheters

13 What are the other nurses in the ward doing?
14 What is the doctor doing?
15 What is one nurse taking?
16 What is the physiotherapist doing?

B

Read through the text and underline all the words and phrases that tell us 'when' something happens.

Something about verbs

1
The simple present tense is used for permanent truths, habitual actions and states.

Water freezes at 32° Fahrenheit.

The sun rises in the morning and sets in the evening.

He smokes a pipe.

It is used with such words as:

usually, generally, often, sometimes, frequently, rarely, never, always, normally, seldom, regularly

and such phrases as:

every day, every week, once a day, once a week, twice a month, several times a year

2
The continuous present tense is used for actions which are going on at the time of speaking. It is usually used without any adverbs of time.

What are you doing? I'm writing a letter.

I'm trying to do these exercises.

It is sometimes used with such words as:

now, still, at present, at the moment

3
The simple past is used for actions which took place in the past and are finished by the time of speaking. It is also used for habitual actions and states in the past, in the same way as the simple present is used for habitual actions and states in the present.

Last year I studied medicine.

I always went to France for my holidays.

She was on an early shift every day last month.

It is used with such words as:

yesterday, last night, the other day, a few days ago, last week, last month, a few moments ago, a long time ago

Drill 1 Simple Past

Jane goes on duty at 7 a.m.	Yesterday – *Jane went on duty at 7 a.m. yesterday.*
The doctor is doing a ward round.	Yesterday – *The doctor did a ward round yesterday.*

1 Jane has to work late. Yesterday –
2 We are very tired. Yesterday –
3 They come off duty at 10 p.m. Yesterday –
4 She is off duty until 2 p.m. Yesterday –
5 I have to go on duty at 7. Yesterday –
6 She is taking a patient to the x-ray department. Yesterday –
7 She is giving a patient a bedpan. Yesterday –
8 They are giving injections. Yesterday –
9 He is taking Mr Smith to the E.N.T. ward. Yesterday –
10 You nurse pneumonia patients. Yesterday –

Drill 2 Questions in the Simple Past

Ask if he went home.	*Did he go home?*
Ask if she did her training here.	*Did she do her training here?*

1 Ask if Jane came on duty at 2 p.m.
2 Ask if she passed her state finals.
3 Ask if she qualified last year.
4 Ask if she gave Mr Jones an injection.
5 Ask if they learned to set trolleys.
6 Ask if she fetched the sterile dressing packs.
7 Ask if she worked in the occupational therapy department.
8 Ask if she assisted Dr Brown.
9 Ask if she found out who he was.
10 Ask if she gave him an injection.

Drill 3 Present Continuous

She always helps the staff nurse.	At the moment – *At the moment she is helping the staff nurse.*
We usually walk past the theatre.	Today – *Today we are walking past the theatre.*

1	She usually works in the E.N.T. ward.	This month –
2	He sometimes assists me.	Now –
3	They carry out sterile procedures.	At the moment –
4	I attend lectures on physiology.	This week –
5	We administer drugs.	Today –
6	She learns to nurse pneumonia-patients.	This week –
7	He shows her the way to the C.S.S.D.	Now –
8	They give urinals and bedpans to bed-patients.	At the moment –
9	She assists the physiotherapist.	This week –
10	They study hard.	Now –

Drill 4 Questions in the Present Continuous

Ask if Jane is training at St. Peter's.	*Is Jane training at St. Peter's?*
Ask if they are working in a medical ward.	*Are they working in a medical ward?*

1 Ask if she is learning to set trolleys.
2 Ask if the physiotherapist is helping this patient.
3 Ask if he is going to the E.N.T. clinic.
4 Ask if the staff nurse is administering drugs.
5 Ask if Jane and Joan are giving injections.
6 Ask if the patients are suffering from cerebral haemorrhage.
7 Ask if this patient is suffering from pneumonia.
8 Ask if he is fetching the sterile dressing packs.
9 Ask if she is taking a patient to the x-ray department.
10 Ask if the sister is talking to the students.

C

Put the verbs in brackets into the correct present or past tense

Notice that, in some of the sentences, time-phrases indicate which tense to use.

Jane and Joan (be) .... both nurses. They (work) ....

at Saint Peter's Hospital. Joan is a qualified nurse. Last year she (pass) .... her State Finals. Jane (train) .... still .... Last month she (work) .... in a medical ward, where she (learn) .... to nurse patients suffering from cardiac infarction and cerebral haemorrhage. She (help) .... the staff nurse, who (explain) .... to her the action, side effects and doses of the drugs. This month Jane (work) .... in one of the hospital's surgical wards. She (learn) .... to set trolleys for sterile procedures. Sometimes she (carry out) .... the procedures herself and sometimes she (assist) .... the doctors. From time to time, she (take) .... patients to the x-ray department or to the physiotherapy department. She often (have) .... to go to the C.S.S.D. to fetch sterile dressing packs. At the moment, she (help) .... another nurse to give a bed-patient a bed-bath. Yesterday she (assist) .... Nurse Brown with t.p.rs. Every day last week, Jane (take) .... the bus to work. She (be) .... on an early shift. She (go) .... on duty at 7 a.m. and (come) .... off duty at 3 p.m. When she is on a late shift, she usually (walk) .... to the hospital. She generally (meet) .... Joan at the bus stop and they (walk) .... to work together. Today Joan is going by bus and Jane (walk) .... to work alone. The sun (shine) .... so Jane (not, carry) .... her umbrella. Last week she (carry) .... her umbrella every day because the weather (be) .... bad.

5 — Sterile Procedures

A central sterile supply department is provided in most modern hospitals. The basic equipment for sterile procedures is obtained in sterile packs from the C.S.S.D. Disposable equipment is often contained in these packs, and, after use, is discarded. Non-disposable equipment is sent back to the C.S.S.D. for re-sterilization.

The following items are normally included in the basic dressing pack: four cotton wool swabs, two dressing towels, four pieces of folded gauze and two gallipots. Sometimes the necessary surgical instruments are included in the dressing pack, sometimes they are supplied in separate packs. A pair of scissors and four pairs of plain dressing forceps or dissecting forceps are generally needed for ward dressings.

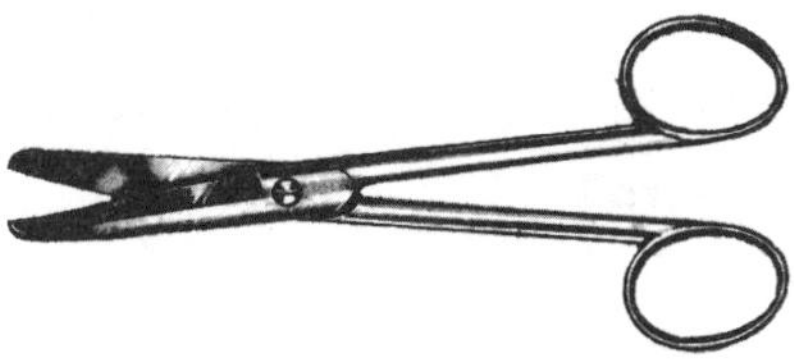

scissors

plain dissecting forceps

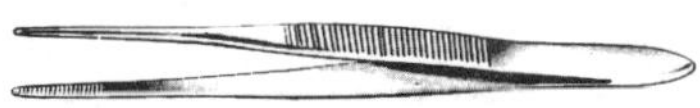

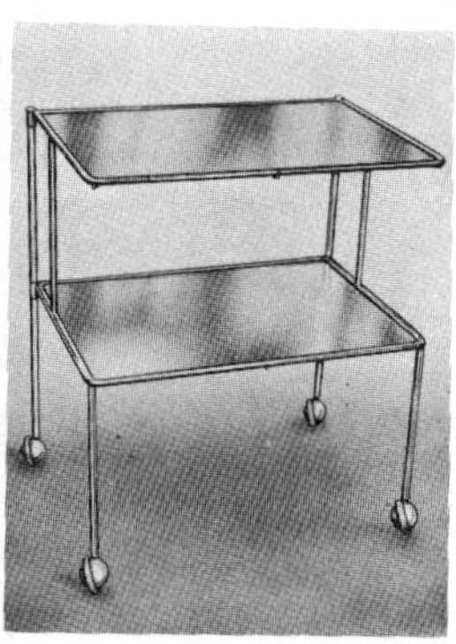

The dressing trolley and how it is prepared

The trolley is washed with soap and water or mopped with an antiseptic such as Sudol. It is then dried. The sterile equipment is put on the top shelf, and the unsterile equipment is put on the bottom shelf.

Top shelf

Sterile pack or bowl containing dressings
Sterile gallipots
Sterile pack or box containing instruments
Jar or cylinder containing instrument handling forceps

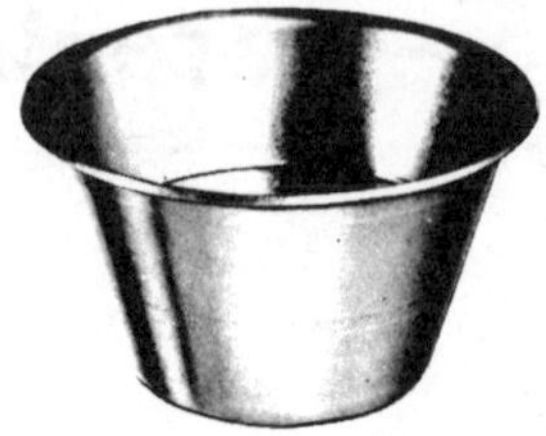

gallipot

Bottom shelf

Bandage tray
Bottles containing antiseptics
Jar or cylinder for used instruments
Paper container for soiled dressings

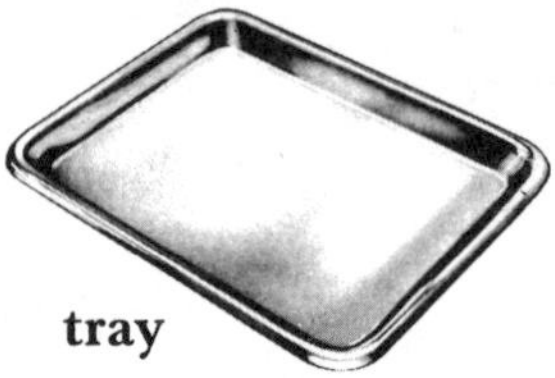

tray

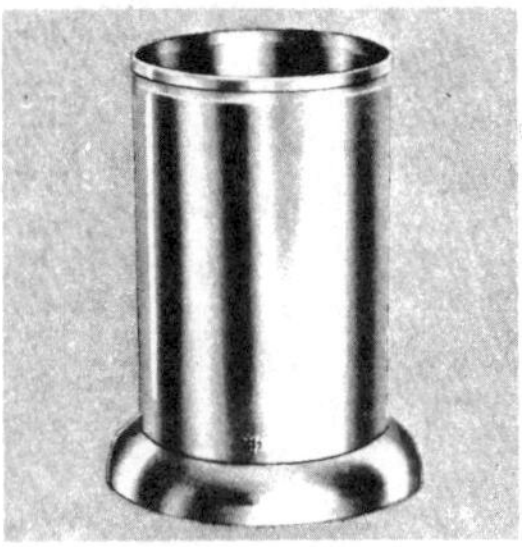

cylinder

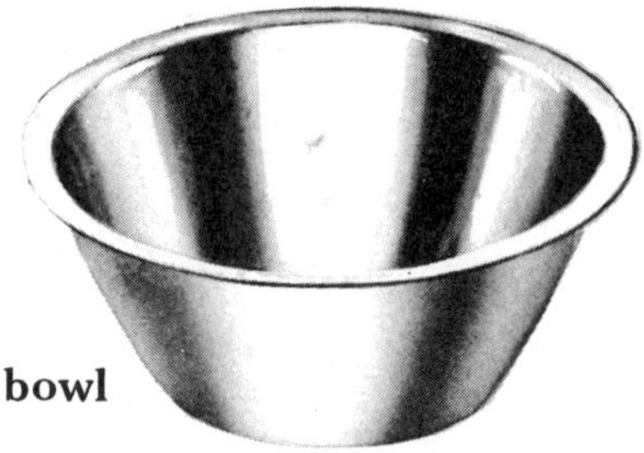

bowl

Some items from the dressing trolley

Cheatle's forceps

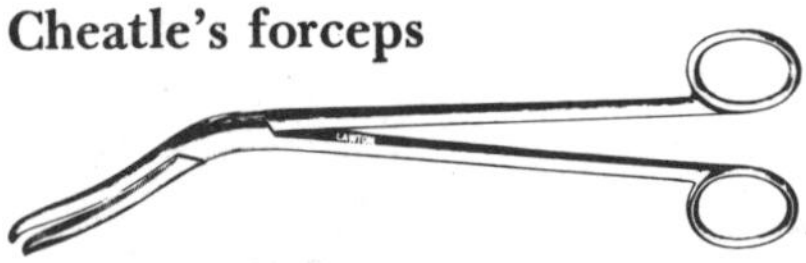

Cheatle's forceps are used for handling sterile instruments. They are sterilized by boiling and placed in a jar containing a suitable disinfectant. The blades and the lower halves of the handles are immersed in the disinfectant.

The bandage tray contains a selection of bandages, adhesive strapping, Nobecutane, a pair of bandage scissors, safety-pins and bandage clips.

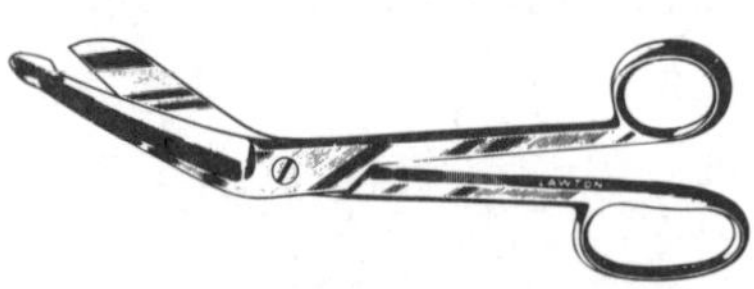

Lister's bandage scissors

The lotion bottles contain Cetrimide or Hibitane for cleaning the skin, and methylated ether for removing Nobecutane or marks left by adhesive tape.

The jar for used instruments contains a suitable disinfectant. Lysol 1 in 40 is often used.

If stitches are to be removed, a pair of sterile suture scissors is added to the basic dressing equipment. If clips are to be removed, a pair of sterile clip-removing forceps is added.

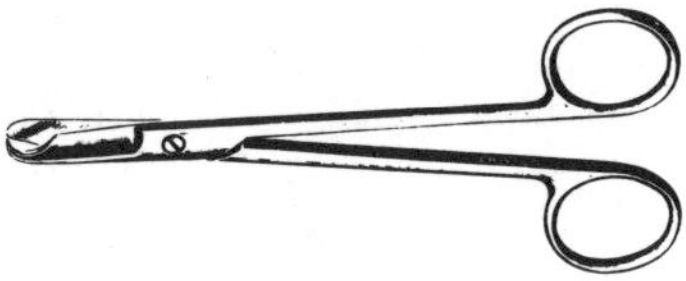

suture scissors

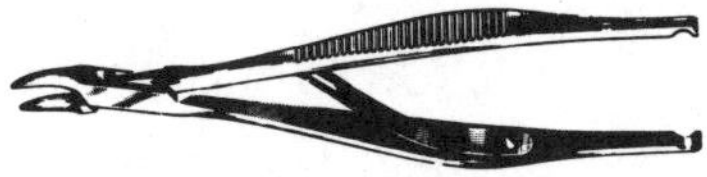

Michel's clip-removing forceps

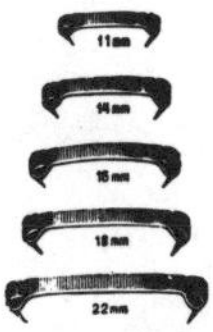

Michel's clips

If a wound is to be explored, sterile ribbon gauze, a sterile wound probe and a pair of sterile sinus forceps are added to the basic equipment.

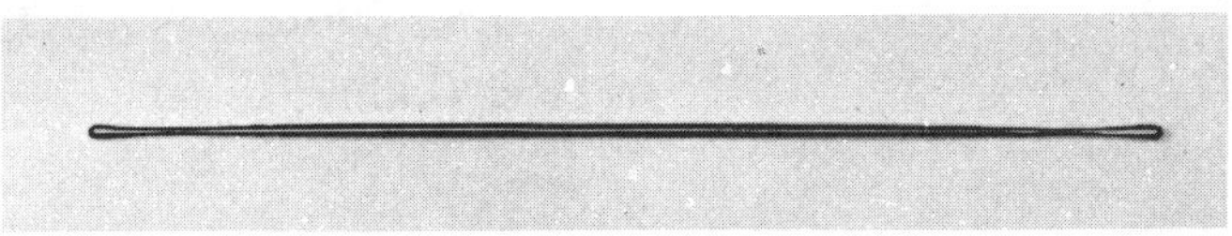

wound probe

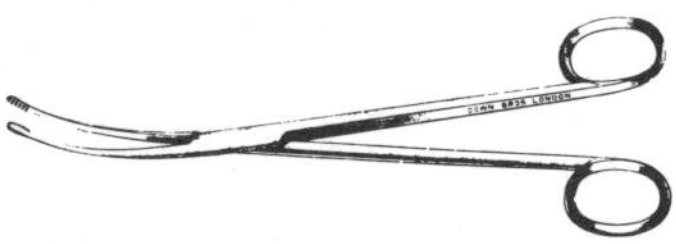

Lister's curved sinus forceps

A

Answer the following questions

1 From where do the wards obtain sterile equipment?
2 What happens to disposable equipment after it is used?
3 What happens to non-disposable equipment after it is used?
4 What items are included in a basic dressing pack?
5 What are dressing trolleys mopped with?
6 What is placed on the top shelf of a dressing trolley?
7 What is placed on the bottom shelf?
8 How are Cheatle's forceps usually sterilized?
9 What does the bandage tray contain?
10 What is methylated ether used for?
11 What does the used instrument jar contain?
12 Where are soiled dressings put?

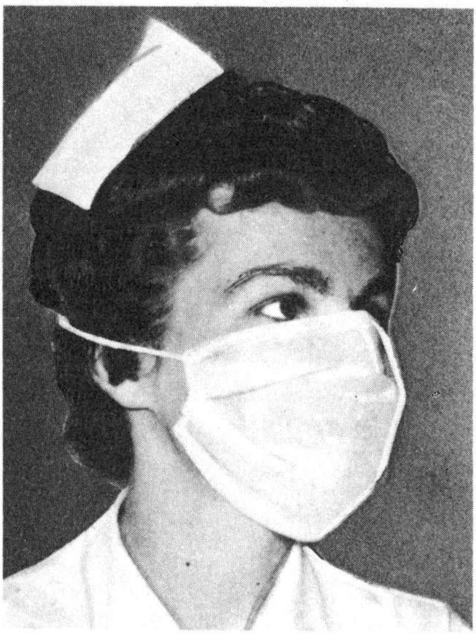

mask

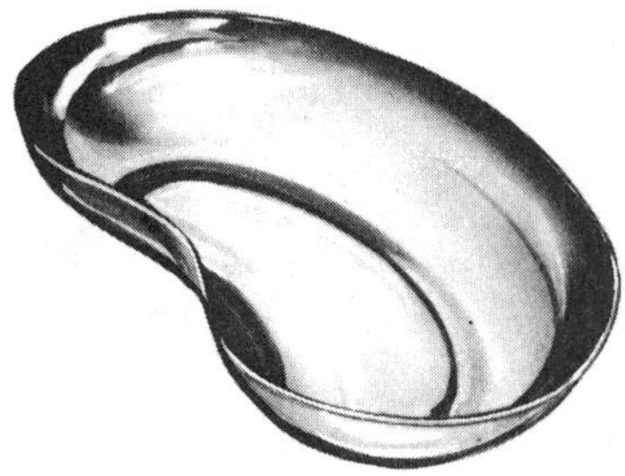

receiver (kidney dish)

More about verbs

Regular verbs

[-t]		[-d]		[-id]
Ache	Stop	Administer	Raise	Assist
Ask	Touch	Breathe	Remember	Attend
Dress	Undress	Bruise	Roll	Discard
Fetch	Walk	Carry	Sprain	Dissect
Finish	Wash	Catheterize	Stay	Fold
Help	Work	Contain	Sterilize	Include
Learn		Dry	Straighten	Need
Look		Explain	Study	Provide
Mop		Lower	Suffer	Want
Nurse		Obtain	Train	
Pass		Open	Try	
Place		Prepare	Turn	
Smoke		Qualify	Use	

Irregular verbs

Be	was/were	been
Bend	bent	bent
Become	became	become
Come	came	come
Cut	cut	cut
Do	did	done
Find	found	found
Freeze	froze	frozen
Get	got	got
Give	gave	given
Go	went	gone
Have	had	had
Hurt	hurt	hurt
Lie	lay	lain
Put	put	put
Rise	rose	risen
See	saw	seen
Send	sent	sent
Set	set	set
Shine	shone	shone
Show	showed	shown
Speak	spoke	spoken
Stand	stood	stood
Take	took	taken

The passive

Look at these sentences, which are all in the present tense.

The basic equipment *is obtained* from the C.S.S.D.

The following items *are included* in the dressing pack.

Non-disposable equipment *is sent* back to the C.S.S.D.

Forceps *are* generally *needed* for ward dressings.

B

What can you say about the trolleys which someone washes with soap and water every day?

The trolleys .... *with soap and water every day.*

What can you say about the equipment which some people send back to the C.S.S.D.?

The equipment .... *back to the C.S.S.D.*

Put the following sentences into the present passive

1 Someone washes the trolley with soap and water.
2 Someone washes the trolleys with soap and water.
3 Someone then dries the trolleys.
4 Someone gives the patient an injection every morning.
5 Someone gives these patients injections every afternoon.
6 Someone discards the disposable equipment after use.
7 Someone carries out most of these procedures in the ward.
8 Someone mops the trolley with an antiseptic.

C

Look at these sentences, which are all in the past tense:

The dressing trolley *was washed* yesterday morning.

The soiled dressings *were discarded*.

Mr Smith *was taken* to the casualty department.

His clothes *were removed*.

Put the following sentences into the past passive

1 Someone took Mr Smith to the orthopaedic ward last night.
2 Someone told them to roll up their sleeves.
3 Someone asked her to take a deep breath.
4 Someone wheeled the trolleys into the ward.
5 Someone performed the operation last week.
6 Someone removed her stitches yesterday morning.
7 Someone gave the baby an injection.
8 Someone admitted Mr and Mrs Jones the day before yesterday.

D

Complete the following sentences with the correct past or present passive forms of the verbs in brackets

1 These patients (catheterize) .... yesterday morning.

2 Mr Smith (give) .... an injection every four hours.

3 These jobs (do) .... usually .... by the student nurses.

4 After the dressings were carried out, the non-disposable equipment (send) .... back to the C.S.S.D.

5 These instruments (need) .... for surgical dressings.

6 Many sterile procedures (carry out) .... in the ward.

7 She (ask) .... to go on duty at 6.30 a.m. yesterday.

8 Disposable equipment (discard) .... after use.

9 Those instruments (discard) .... yesterday.

10 The patient (help) .... into bed.

E

Complete the following sentences with the correct word from this list

on, by, as, from, back, off, up, of, in, for, to, with, down, out, against

1 He's got a pain .... his chest.

2 Would you lie .... the examination couch, please?

3 She works .... a surgical ward.

4 They always go .... work .... bus.

5 When she's .... an early shift, she goes .... duty at 7 a.m.

6 This morning we are attending lectures .... physiology and hygiene.

7 This patient has a rash .... his stomach.

8 Mary is now working .... a staff nurse in an ear, nose and throat ward.

9 Jane is learning to set trolleys .... sterile procedures.

10 This patient is suffering .... cerebral haemorrhage.

11 The sister is explaining .... the students the doses of various drugs.

12 This equipment is obtained .... the C.S.S.D.

13 The trolleys are mopped .... an antiseptic.

14 Sterile equipment is placed .... the top shelf .... the trolley.

15 Sterile instruments are handled .... Cheatle's forceps.

16 Ask the patient to roll .... his sleeve, please.

17 Ask Mr Smith to take .... his shirt, please.

18 Now ask him to put it .... again.

6 — Instruments

Last week, Joan tested Jane on instruments. They had a pile of pictures in front of them. Sometimes Joan held up a picture and asked Jane to name it. Sometimes Joan said the name of an instrument and Jane had to find the correct picture. This was the first picture

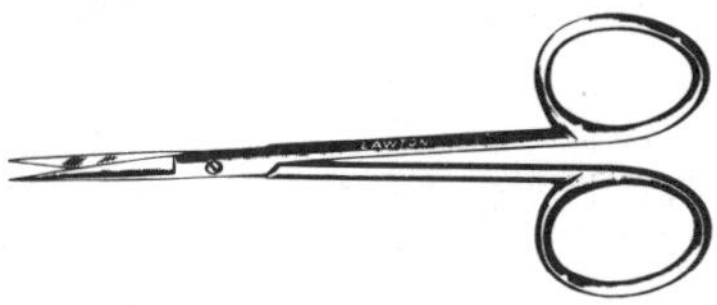

and Jane said, "Easy, they're scissors."

"But what shape are they?" asked Joan.

"Well, they're straight."

"Now look at the blades."

"They're sharp-ended," answered Jane.

"Good," said Joan, "they're straight, sharp-ended scissors. What about these, then?"

And Joan held up this picture:

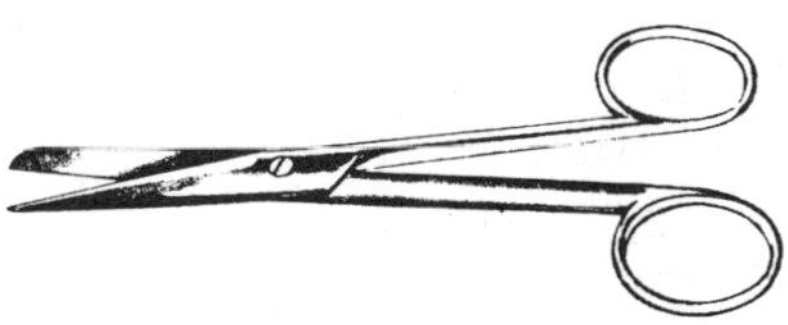

Jane sighed. "Those, my dear Joan, are a pair of straight, sharp- and blunt-ended scissors."

What do you think Jane said for this picture?

(a)

"They're ...."

Joan agreed, but said, "What type are they?"

"They're ....

...."

"And what type of scissors are these?"

(b)

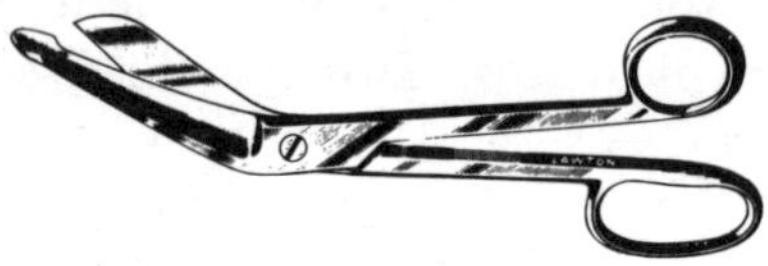

"They're ....

...."

Next, Joan held up two pictures at once and asked, "What are these two?"

(c)

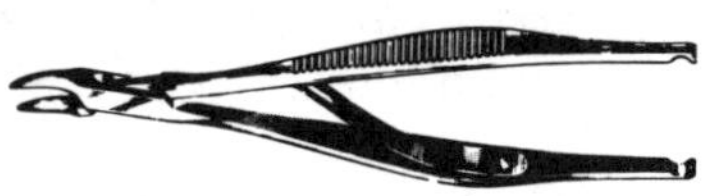

"Those are ....

....

(d)

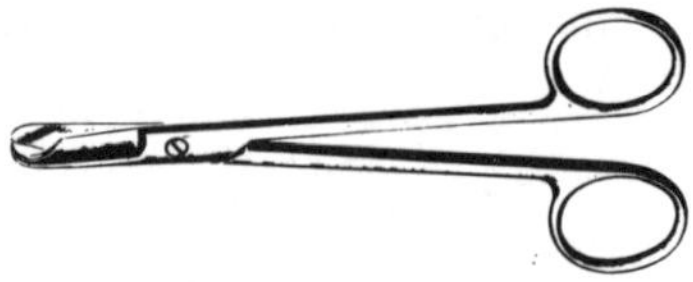

and those are ....

..............................," answered Jane.

Then Joan showed Jane some more pictures of a lot more instruments. One was of a *straight* instrument, like this

(e)

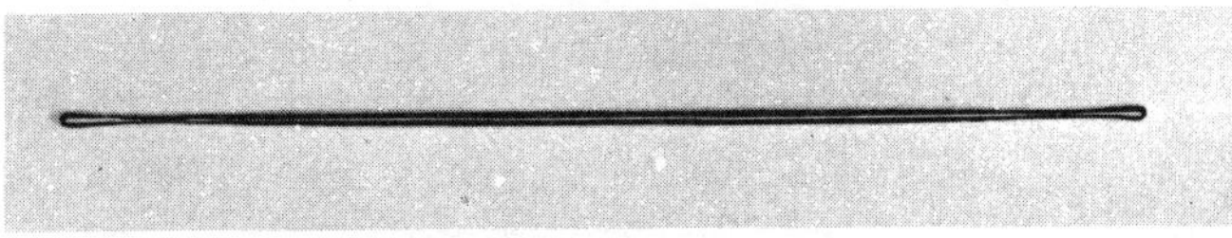

"It's a ...."

Another was of a *curved* one, like this

(f)

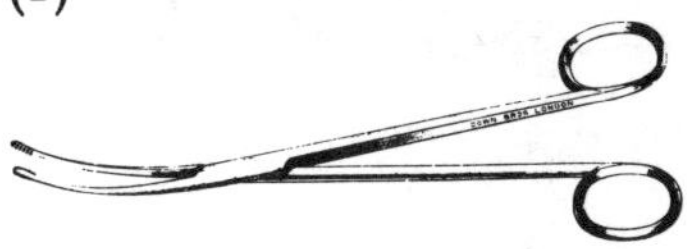

"They're ....

....................................."

And a third was of an *angular* instrument

(g)

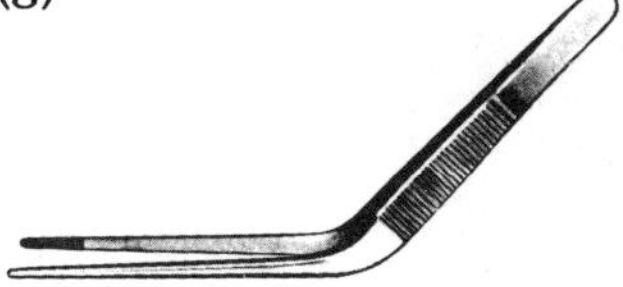

"They're ....

....................................."

On the next pages, there are pictures of other instruments on which Joan tested Jane. Not to worry; Jane didn't get them all right, and Joan had to tell her.

A

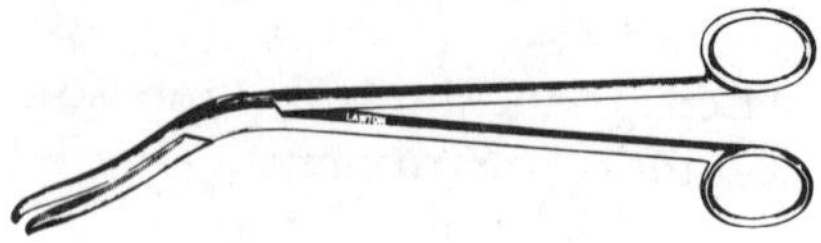

1 They're ....

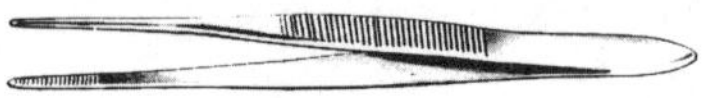

2 They're ....

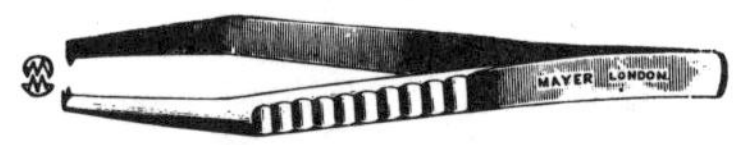

3 They're ....

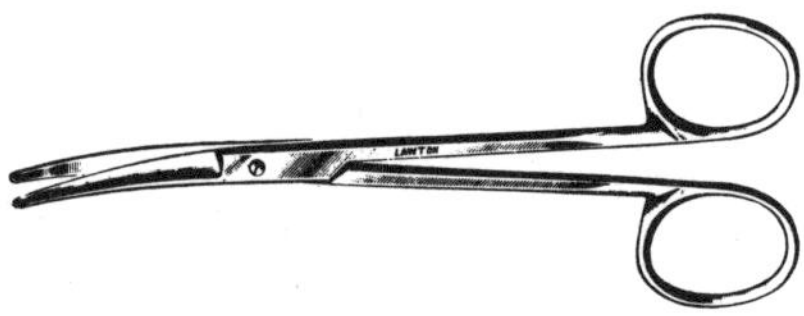

4 They're ....

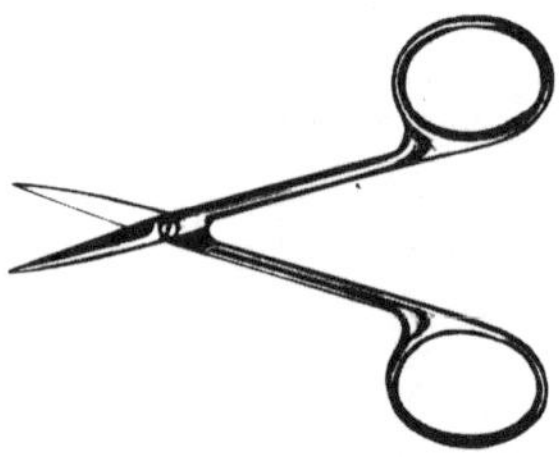

5 They're ....

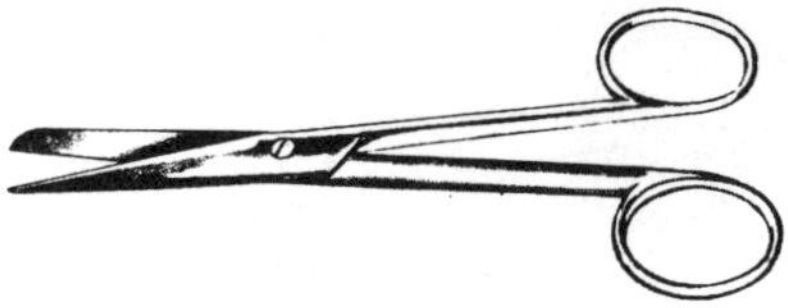

6 They're ....

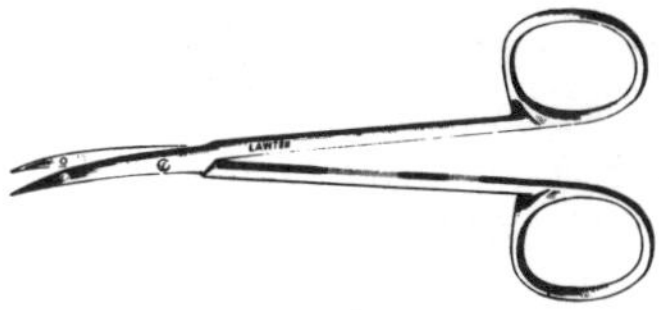

7 They're ....

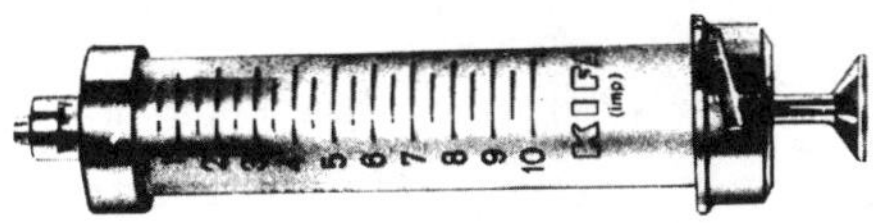

8 It's a ....

9 It's a ....

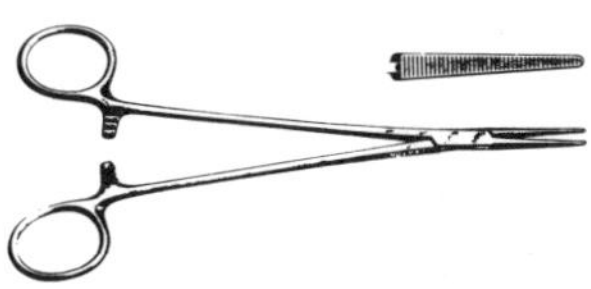

10 They're ....

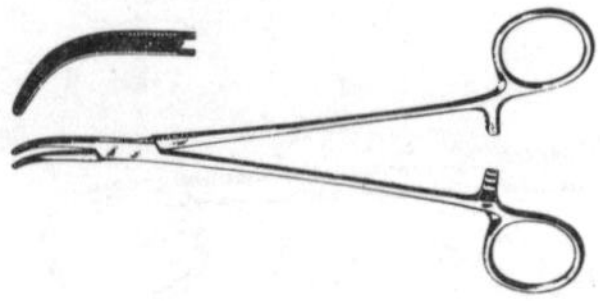

11 They're ....

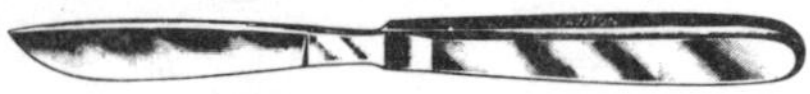

12 It's a ....

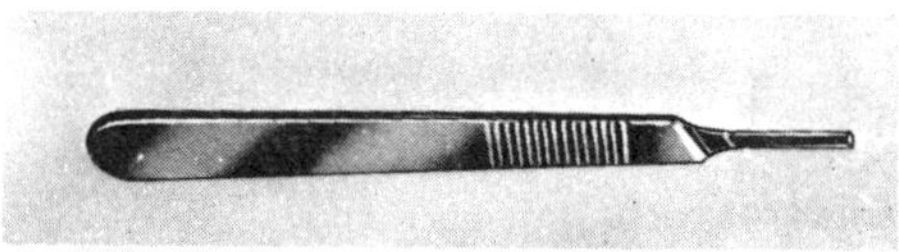

13 It's a ....

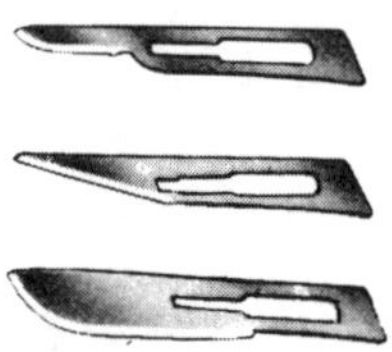

14 They're ....

B

Which instruments are used

1 for taking out stitches?
2 for giving injections?
3 for exploring a wound?
4 for handling sterile dressings?
5 for cutting bandages?
6 for removing clips?
7 for stopping bleeding?
8 for handling sterile instruments?

C

1 A wound probe and sinus forceps are used for .... a wound.

2 Cheatle's forceps are used for .... sterile instruments.

3 Artery forceps are used for .... bleeding.

4 A syringe and needle are used for .... injections.

5 Bandage scissors are used for .... bandages.

6 Dissecting forceps are used for .... sterile dressings.

7 Suture scissors are used for .... sutures.

8 Clip-removing forceps are used for .... clips.

D

Instead of saying, "You use suture scissors *for removing* stitches," you can say, "You use suture scissors *to remove* stitches."

Look at these examples and rewrite the following sentences in the passive:

You use suture scissors to remove stitches.
Suture scissors are used to remove stitches.

You use Hibitane to clean the skin.
Hibitane is used to clean the skin.

1 You use Cheatle's forceps to handle sterile instruments.
2 You use Michel's clip-removing forceps to remove clips.
3 You use methylated ether to remove Nobecutane.
4 You use wound probes to explore wounds.
5 You use a syringe to give injections.
6 You use artery forceps to stop bleeding.
7 You use dissecting forceps to handle sterile dressings.
8 You use a thermometer to take temperatures.

E

Vocabulary

1 We can talk about instrument handling forceps or ....

2 We can say The blades and the lower halves of the handles are covered by the disinfectant or

They are .... the disinfectant.

3 We can say There is a selection of bandages in the bandage tray or

The bandage tray .... a selection of bandages.

4 We can talk about stitches or ....

5 We can talk about things that are used once and then thrown away or

....

6 We can say small bowls or ....

7 We can say some scissors or ....

8 We can say They are provided in separate packs or

They are .... in separate packs.

9 We can talk about taking away marks left by adhesive tape or

.... marks left by adhesive tape.

10 We can talk about a round glass container or a ....

7 — Disinfectants and Antiseptics

Disinfectants are toxic chemical substances which destroy micro-organisms and living tissue. Antiseptics are less toxic substances which inhibit the growth of micro-organisms. Generally speaking, disinfectants are used for sterilizing inanimate objects, and antiseptics are used for cleansing the skin and maintaining the sterility of boiled or autoclaved instruments. These definitions are, however, not precise because the destructive power of a disinfectant depends on its strength and the length of time for which it is used. Nowadays, disinfectants are often referred to as 'bactericides' because they kill bacteria, and antiseptics are called 'bacteriostatics' because they prevent bacteria from growing and multiplying.

Some chemical agents commonly used as disinfectants or antiseptics

Substance	*Use*
Proflavine	for disinfecting the skin and swabbing wounds
Gentian violet	for preparing the skin before operation
Tincture of iodine	for disinfecting the skin
Cetrimide	for disinfecting the skin, instruments and other equipment
Hydrogen peroxide	for irrigating wounds and cavities and removing pus and blood
Hibitane	for disinfecting the skin and instruments
Lysol	for disinfecting floors, baths, clothes etc.
Phenol	for disinfecting linen sanitary equipment and excreta

A

Answer these questions

1 What do disinfectants do?

2 What do antiseptics do?

3 What are disinfectants used for?

4 What are antiseptics used for?

5 What does the destructive power of a disinfectant depend on?

6 Why are disinfectants sometimes called bactericides?

7 Why are antiseptics sometimes called bacteriostatics?

B

Vocabulary

1	We can say	Lysol is a poisonous substance or Lysol is a .... substance.
2	Instead of saying	Micro-organisms are killed by disinfectants, we can say, Micro-organisms are .... disinfectants.
3	We can say	Antiseptics prevent bacteria from growing and multiplying or Antiseptics .... the growth of bacteria.
4	We can talk about	objects that are not alive or ....
5	We can say	Hydrogen peroxide is used for washing out wounds and cavities or Hydrogen peroxide is used for .... wounds and cavities.
6	We can talk about	preserving the sterility of equipment or .... the sterility of equipment.
7	We can say	Instruments are sterilized by steam under pressure or Instruments are sterilized by ....
8	One word for	urine, faeces and sputum is ....
9	We can talk about	antiseptics or ...., and disinfectants or ....
10	Instead of saying	An exact definition, we can say, A .... definition.
11	We can talk about	cleaning the skin or .... the skin.
12	We can talk about	a chemical agent or a chemical ....

C

Look at the examples and rewrite the following sentences as questions

Proflavine is used for swabbing wounds.
Is Proflavine used for swabbing wounds?

Hibitane and Cetrimide are used for disinfecting the skin.
Are Hibitane and Cetrimide used for disinfecting the skin?

1 Methylated ether is used to remove Nobecutane.
2 Disinfectants are used to disinfect inanimate objects.
3 Hydrogen peroxide is used for irrigating cavities.
4 Gentian violet is used for preparing the skin before operation.
5 Phenol is used to disinfect excreta.
6 Cetrimide is used for swabbing wounds.
7 Sinus forceps are used to explore wounds.
8 Thermometers are used for taking temperatures.

D

Look at the examples and rewrite the following sentences correctly in the negative

Dressing trolleys are mopped with ether.
Dressing trolleys aren't mopped with ether.

A catheter is used to take temperatures.
A catheter isn't used to take temperatures.

1 Maternity cases are nursed in geriatric wards.
2 Tincture of iodine is used for removing pus and blood.
3 Antiseptics are used for sterilizing inanimate objects.
4 Disinfectants are called bacteriostatics.
5 Non-disposable equipment is thrown away after use.
6 Drugs are obtained from the physiotherapy department.
7 Operations are carried out in the dispensary.
8 Clip-removing forceps are used to take out sutures.

8 — Casualty 1

While John Smith was going to school this morning, a car knocked him down. His right leg was broken just below the knee. Some people who saw the accident laid him in a comfortable position on the pavement and telephoned for an ambulance. John was badly shocked and in great pain. While the people were waiting for the ambulance, the driver of the car that knocked John down covered him with a coat and tried to comfort him.

When the ambulance arrived, John was lifted onto a stretcher, put into the ambulance and driven to a hospital that was not far away. When he arrived at the casualty department, he was admitted. The nurse who admitted him gave him an injection of morphine to combat the shock and the pain. The doctor who examined him comforted him and told him everything would be all right. While the doctor was examining him, the nurse who had admitted him took his pulse and blood pressure. No anti-tetanus injection was necessary as John had been immunized against tetanus six months earlier.

As John's wound was lacerated and contused, he was given an antibiotic to prevent the onset of infection. He was then taken to the x-ray department. While the x-ray examination was being carried out, John's parents arrived at the hospital. The doctor who examined John told them that John had sustained a compound fracture of the tibia and fibula. He explained that an operation was necessary and asked Mr Smith to sign a consent for operation form. Mr Smith signed the consent form while Mrs Smith was giving John's personal particulars and previous medical history to the nurse. Before John's parents left the hospital, they were told when they could visit him and were given a list of things that he would need.

While John was waiting to go to theatre, a quarter-hourly record of his pulse and blood pressure was kept and he was given a suitable premedication.

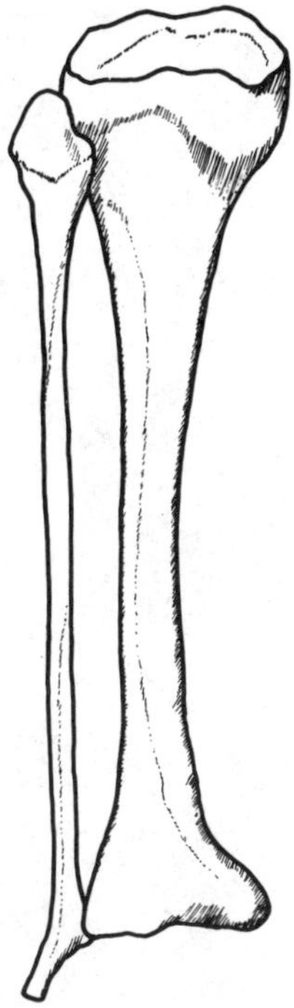

anterior aspect, right tibia and fibula

CAMBURY GENERAL HOSPITAL

NAME	WARD/DEPT.	HOSP. REG. No.

I ______________________________

of ______________________________

hereby consent to undergo the operation of ______________________________
the effect and nature of which has been explained to me.

I also consent to such further or alternative operative measures as may be found to be necessary during the course of such operation, and to the administration of a local or other anaesthetic for the purpose of the same.

I understand that an assurance has not been given that the operation will be performed by a particular surgeon.

Dated this ______________ day of ______________

(Signed) ______________________________

OPERATION CONSENT (PATIENT)

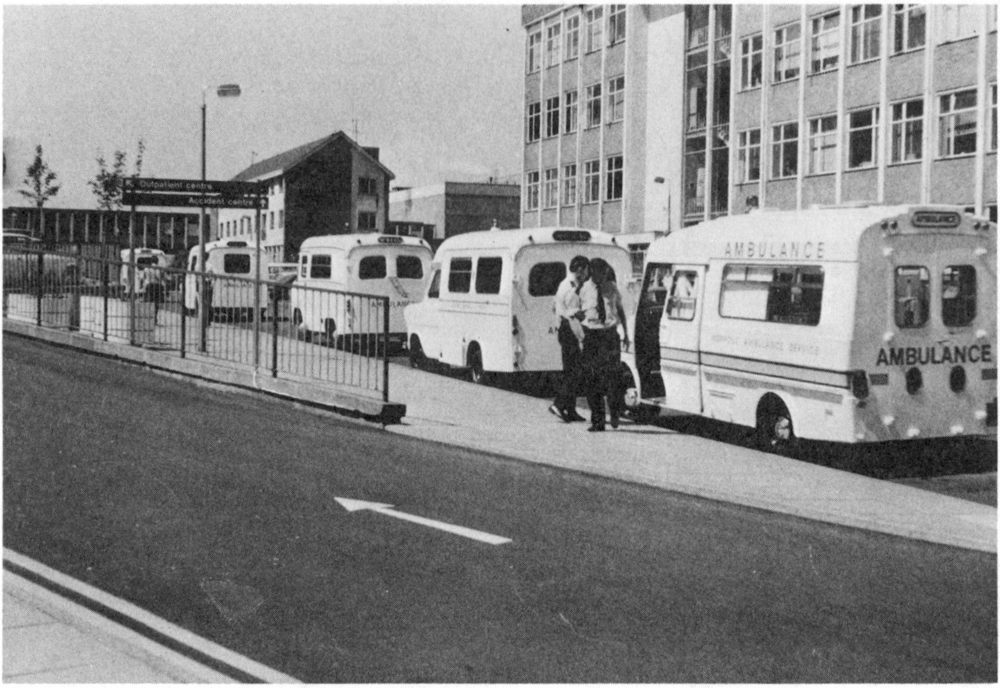

Ambulances outside Addenbrooke's Hospital, Cambridge

A

Answer the following questions

1 What was John doing when he was knocked down?
2 What did the people who saw the accident do?
3 What did the driver of the car that knocked John down do?
4 What happened when the ambulance arrived?
5 Who gave him an injection of morphine?
6 Why was he given morphine?
7 Why wasn't he given an anti-tetanus injection?
8 What sort of wound had John sustained?
9 Which bones had been broken?
10 What was Mr Smith asked to sign?
11 What was Mrs Smith asked to give?
12 What record was kept while he was waiting to go to theatre?

B

Read the text carefully. Then fill in the blanks with suitable words

Do not look at the text again until you have tried to complete all the sentences.

John was k............ d........... by a car. Some people who saw the a............... called for help. John was badly s.................. and in great p............ Someone covered him with a c.............. When the a...................... arrived, John was lifted onto a s................... He was taken to the c............. d....... .... of the local hospital. He was given an i..................... to combat the s............ and the p.......... John's wound was l................. and c...................... He had sustained a c.................. f.................... of the t......... and f............ Mrs Smith gave John's personal p.................. and previous m............... h................ While John was waiting to go to theatre, he was given a suitable p...................

Relatives

Who and that

Look at these sentences

Some people *who* saw the accident called the ambulance.
The driver of the car *that* knocked him down waited for the police.
The nurse *who* admitted him gave him an injection of morphine.
He was driven to a hospital *that* was not far away.

In the sentences above we have used 'who' for people, and 'that' for things.

C

Complete the following sentences with 'who' or 'that'

1 The ambulance .... took John to hospital was driven by Mr Brown.

2 Nurses .... carry out sterile procedures must wash their hands thoroughly before they begin.

3 The radiographer .... x-rayed John tried to comfort him.

4 The dry dressing .... covered John's wound was sterile.

5 Disinfectants are chemical substances .... destroy bacteria.

6 He was given a premedication .... dried up his secretions.

7 The surgeon .... performed the operation was from Germany.

8 The nurse .... kept a record of John's pulse and blood pressure was Jane Johnson.

9 John was given an injection .... relieved his pain.

10 The hospital .... is outside Cambury is Cambury General.

11 The doctor .... explained that an operation was necessary asked Mr Smith to sign a consent form.

12 People .... cross the road without looking are fools.

The Past Continuous Tense

Active

I He She It	was	going coming having running
You We They	were	calling watching assisting

Passive

I He She It	was	being	lifted driven assisted used
You We They	were		taken carried given

The past continuous tense is used

1 When two actions were happening at the same time in the past:

Jane was scrubbing the floor while Mary was cleaning the window.
Some patients were watching TV while others were playing chess.

2 When one action in the past (usually a longer one) is interrupted by another (usually a shorter one):

While John was going to school this morning, a car knocked him down.
When the accident happened, Mary was standing at the bus stop.

Here 'when' refers to action at a point of time and 'while' to action during a period of time.

D
Complete the following sentences with the past continuous tense

1 The children (play) .... in the street.

2 When the telephone rang, I (read) .... the newspaper.

3 We (sit) .... in the garden when it started to rain.

4 I (write) .... a letter while my sister was reading a book.

5 You (go) .... to work when the accident happened.

E
Complete the following sentences with the correct past simple or past continuous tense of the verbs in brackets

1 While John (lie) .... on the pavement, somebody (call) .... for an ambulance.

2 Mary (see) .... the accident while she (wait) .... for the bus.

3 I (read) .... a book when the telephone (ring) ....

4 John (lie) .... in hospital when his parents (arrive) ....

5 Mr Smith (sign) .... the consent for operation form while Mrs Smith (talk) .... to the nurse.

6 Jane (meet) .... Joan while she (train) .... at St. Peter's.

7 When the staff nurse (come) .... on duty, Jane (give) .... Mr Brown a bed-bath.

8 While the patients (have) .... breakfast, the night sister (go) .... off duty.

9 John (be given) .... a premedication while he (wait) .... to go to theatre.

10 Joan (set) .... a trolley when the new patient (be admitted) ....

11 While she (go) .... to the occupational therapy department, she (see) .... the ambulance.

12 While the x-ray examination (be carried out) ...., John's parents (arrive) .... at the hospital.

13 When it (start) .... to rain, we (sit) .... in the garden.

14 They (meet) .... Mary and Jane outside the main gate while they (wait) .... for Peter and Bob.

9 — Casualty 2

In the theatre, John will be given an anaesthetic and his wound will be explored. The x-rays which were taken by the radiographer will show the surgeon the exact site and extent of the fracture. Dead or dirty tissue will be excised and any small splinters of bone will be removed. The surgeon will perform the operation using a 'no touch' technique to reduce the chances of infection.

When the surgeon is satisfied that the wound is as clean as possible, he will dust it off with an antibiotic powder. He will then suture it and cover it with a sterile gauze dressing. Any areas that are raw will be dressed with sterile Vaseline petroleum jelly gauze. The surgeon will now be able to treat the fracture as closed. He will reduce the bones into their anatomical position, and the leg will be put in plaster of Paris. John will then be taken back to an orthopaedic ward.

*

When a post-operative patient like John arrives in the ward, he is carefully lifted from the stretcher and laid in a specially prepared bed. The foot of the bed is often raised on wooden blocks. The patient is placed on his back with his head turned to one side. As he is generally still unconscious, an artificial airway is in position and a nurse stays with him to ensure that his airway is kept clear. She also checks his pulse rate and volume, his colour and the rate and depth of his respirations.

A

Answer the following questions

1 What will John be given in theatre?
2 What will be done to his wound?
3 What will the x-rays show the surgeon?
4 What will happen to any dead or dirty tissue?
5 What will happen to any small splinters of bone?
6 Why will the surgeon use a 'no touch' technique?

7 What will the surgeon do to the wound when he is satisfied it is as clean as possible?
8 What will he do to the wound when he has sutured it?
9 What will any raw areas be dressed with?
10 What will he do to the fractured bones?
11 What will he do to John's leg?
12 Where will John be taken after the operation?
13 What happens to a post-operative patient when he arrives in the ward?
14 How is he placed in bed?
15 What does he have in his mouth?
16 Why does a nurse remain with him?
17 What does the nurse check?

B

Read the text carefully and complete the following sentences

In the theatre, John will be given an a....................... The x-rays will show the s................. the exact s.......... and e......... of the fracture. Dead or dirty t............... will be excised and any s........................ of bone will be removed. The surgeon will perform the o................. using a 'no touch' t...............

When the surgeon is satisfied that John's w.............. is as clean as possible, he will dust it off with an a.................. powder. It will then be sutured and covered with a sterile g............ d.............

The surgeon will now be able to treat the f................. as closed.

He will reduce the bones into their a................. position, and the leg will be put in p............. of P............ John will then be taken back to an o....................... w...........

When a p........-............... patient arrives in the ward, he is carefully lifted from the s.................. and laid in a specially prepared bed. As he is generally still u...................., an a................ airway is in position and a nurse stays with him to ensure that his a........... is kept clear. She also checks his pulse rate and v.................., his c............. and the rate and d........... of his r..................

C

We can say

1 The surgeon examined John's wound.
or
The surgeon .... John's wound.

2 He cut away the dead tissue.
or
He .... the dead tissue.

3 He took away the small splinters of bone.
or
He .... the small splinters of bone.

4 He carried out the operation.
or
He .... the operation.

5 He used a technique to make the risk of infection smaller.
or
He used a technique to .... the risk of infection.

6 He sewed up the wound.
or
He .... the wound.

7 He replaced the bones in their normal position.
or
He .... the bones .... their ....
....

Relatives

That

In the following examples, 'that' is an object pronoun. It can be used for both people and things, but we prefer to leave it out.

The man (that) you saw yesterday is my uncle.

The man you saw yesterday is my uncle.

The book (that) you are reading is mine.

The book you are reading is mine.

D

Rewrite the following pairs of sentences as one sentence

1 The letter was from Germany. We received it this morning.
2 The doctor has just left. You wanted to see him.
3 The story is very interesting. I've just read it.
4 The instrument is a wound probe. The sister is using it.
5 The nurse comes on duty at 9.30. We saw her yesterday.

E

Complete the following sentences with 'who' or 'that'. Leave out 'that' where possible

1 The nurse .... admitted John gave him an injection.
2 The instrument .... is on the table is a syringe.
3 Only instruments .... have been sterilized are used in this department.
4 The instrument .... the doctor is using is a stethoscope.
5 She is talking to the nurse .... we met last week.
6 The gloves .... she lost were old.
7 The boy .... had the accident was taken to hospital.
8 The girl .... she knocked down was taken to hospital.
9 The girl .... lives near me is a nurse.

The Future Tense

Active

I We	shall	have explore
You He She It They	will	suture examine cover reduce take

Passive

I We	shall	be	taken shown
You He She It They	will		examined x-rayed put covered driven

Nowadays 'shall' and 'will' are almost always shortened to ''ll', 'shall not' to 'shan't' and 'will not' to 'won't'.

F

Complete the following sentences with the future tense, active or passive

1 The anaesthetist (give) .... John an anaesthetic.

2 In theatre, his wound (explore) .... by the surgeon.

3 I (visit) .... John tomorrow afternoon.

4 The surgeon (remove) .... any small splinters of bone.

5 Any dead or dirty tissue (remove) .... by the surgeon.

6 The surgeon (reduce) .... the bones into their anatomical position.

7 When the operation is completed, John (take) .... to an orthopaedic ward.

8 The physiotherapist (see) .... John tomorrow.

9 The patient (not, be) .... conscious when he arrives in the ward.

10 We (go) .... on duty at 9.30 a.m. tomorrow.

Drill 1 Future

I go on duty.	Tomorrow – *I'll go on duty at 7 o'clock.*
She sets a trolley.	Tomorrow – *She'll set a trolley.*

1 He performs the operation. Tomorrow –
2 He examines the patient. Tomorrow –
3 She sterilizes the equipment. Tomorrow –
4 They watch television. Tomorrow –
5 I finish my book. Tomorrow –
6 We visit him at 2.30. Tomorrow –
7 She gives him an injection. Tomorrow –
8 I feel better. Tomorrow –

Drill 2

He is given an anaesthetic.	Tomorrow – *He'll be given an anaesthetic.*
She is taken to theatre.	Tomorrow – *She'll be taken to theatre.*

1 His wound is explored. Tomorrow –
2 Dirty tissue is excised. Tomorrow –
3 We are given an antibiotic. Tomorrow –
4 You are given an anaesthetic. Tomorrow –
5 The patient is taken to x-ray. Tomorrow –
6 We are driven to the hospital. Tomorrow –
7 My arm is put in plaster. Tomorrow –
8 I am sent home. Tomorrow –

Drill 3 Questions

You will go.	Where – *Where'll you go?*
She will see me.	When – *When'll she see me?*
1 She will finish her training.	When –
2 He will have an operation.	When –
3 They will be admitted.	When –
4 He will be given an antibiotic.	Why –
5 We shall go.	Where –
6 I shall do it.	How –
7 We shall meet her.	Where –
8 He will visit them.	When –

Drill 4 Negatives

They will help us.	*They won't help us.*
I shall go.	*I shan't go.*

1 He will leave tomorrow.
2 You will be given an injection.
3 I shall be sent home tomorrow.
4 She will go off duty at six.
5 This will hurt you.
6 Your leg will be put in plaster.
7 An anaesthetic will be necessary.
8 We shall visit him next week.

10 — Casualty 3

Soon after John had returned to the ward, he began to regain consciousness. The nurse who was looking after him removed the airway from his mouth and gave him a pillow for his head. For the next few hours he slept soundly. From time to time the toes of his injured leg were examined to see if they were warm and pink, and his pulse and blood pressure were taken half-hourly.

At 6 p.m. John woke up and complained of severe pain in his leg. The surgeon who had performed the operation had prescribed Pethidine if John complained of pain, and he was given an intramuscular injection of 50 mgs of Pethidine at 6.10 p.m. As his blood pressure was now within normal limits, the bed-blocks were taken away and a bed-cradle was put in his bed to take the weight of the bedclothes off his legs. A nurse offered him a bottle, but he said he could not manage to pass water.

A houseman visited John during the evening to check that he was all right and that he would be able to sleep. He prescribed a second injection of Pethidine, which was to be given at midnight if John complained of further pain. Two nurses came and helped John to wash his hands and face and to change from the white theatre gown into his own pyjama jacket. John, who had been allowed frequent sips of water because he had not complained of nausea, was now given a cup of tea and told the nurses that he was beginning to feel fine.

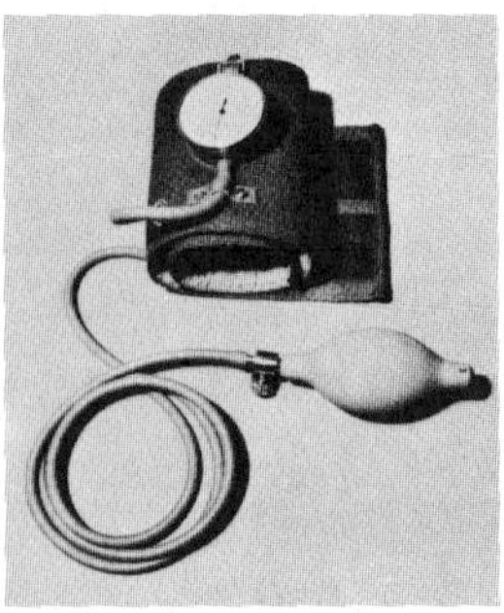

sphygmomanometer

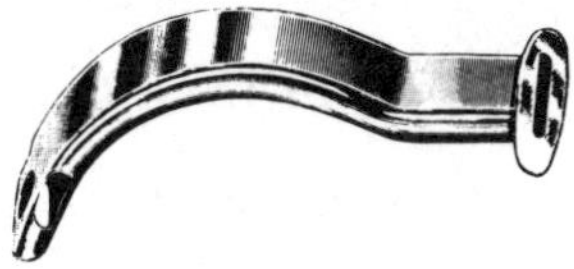

artificial airway

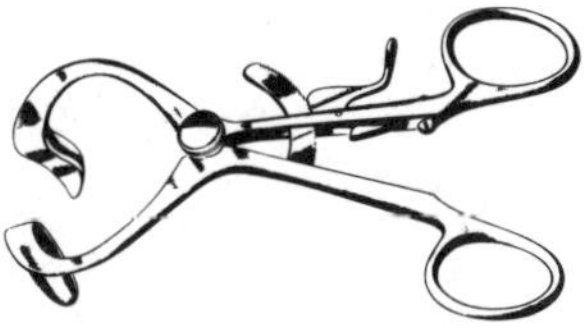

gag

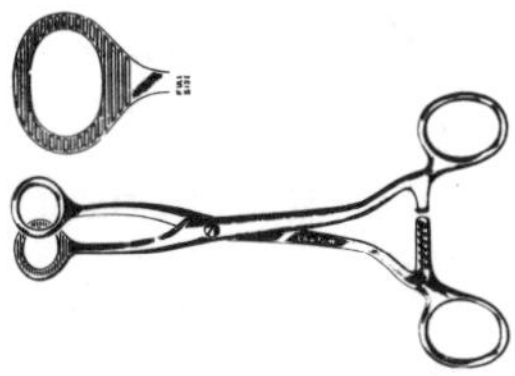

tongue forceps

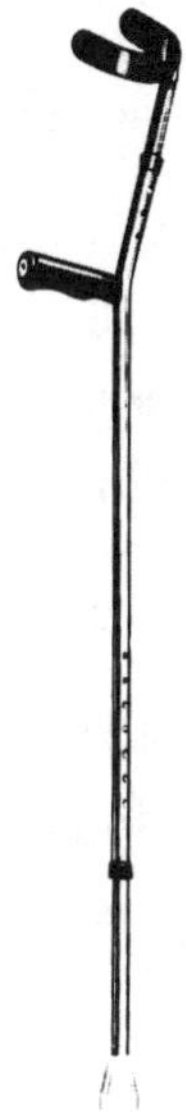

crutch

A

Answer the following questions

1 What happened soon after John returned to the ward?
2 What did the nurse who was looking after him do?
3 What did John do when he woke up at 6 p.m?
4 What was John given at 6.10 p.m?
5 Who had prescribed the Pethidine?
6 Why was a bed-cradle put in John's bed?
7 Why did a houseman visit John during the evening?
8 What did the two nurses help John to do?
9 Had John complained of feeling sick?
10 What did he tell the nurses?

B

Complete the following sentences with words from the list

off, during, from, up, for, of, within, into, away, in

1 A nurse removed the artificial airway .... his mouth.

2 She gave him a pillow .... his head.

3 John woke .... and complained .... severe pain .... his leg.

4 As his blood pressure was now .... normal limits, the bed-blocks were taken ....

5 A bed-cradle was put .... his bed to take the weight .... the bedclothes .... his leg.

6 A houseman visited John .... the evening.

7 Two nurses helped John to change .... the theatre gown ...... his own pyjama jacket.

8 John had been allowed frequent sips .... water because he had not complained .... nausea.

C

Vocabulary

We can say

1 A doctor orders the use of a drug.
or
A doctor .... a drug.

2 The patient is coming round.
or
The patient is ....

3 The patient complained of feeling sick.
or
The patient complained of ....

4 She is sleeping deeply.
or
She is sleeping ....

5 T.p.rs are taken every 30 minutes.
or
T.p.rs are taken ....-.......... .

6 The patient complains of pain again.
or
The patient complains of .... pain.

7 He is complaining of very bad pain.
or
He is complaining of .... pain.

8 The nurse offered him a urinal.
or
The nurse offered him a ....

9 The surgeon who carried out the operation.
or
The surgeon who .... the operation.

10 The artificial airway was taken from his mouth.
or
The artificial airway was .... from his mouth.

D

Put the following sentences into the passive

1 A nurse removed the artificial airway from his mouth.
2 A nurse examined the toes of his injured leg.
3 A nurse took his pulse and blood pressure half-hourly.
4 A nurse gave him a pillow for his head.
5 A nurse gave him an intramuscular injection of Pethidine.
6 A nurse asked Mr and Mrs Smith to come back the next day.
7 A nurse gave John a cup of tea.
8 A nurse offered him a urinal.

Drill 1 Past Passive

The patient is admitted.	Yesterday – *The patient was admitted yesterday.*
The injections are given.	Last night – *The injections were given last night.*

1	His bed-blocks are removed.	Yesterday –
2	The injection is given at 10 o'clock.	Yesterday morning –
3	Her blood pressure is taken four-hourly.	Yesterday –
4	He is examined in the casualty department.	Yesterday evening –
5	They are taken to hospital by ambulance.	Last night –
6	The operation is performed by Mr Jones.	This morning –
7	His parents are asked to sign a consent form.	Last night –
8	The new patient is taken to the x-ray department.	This morning –

Drill 2 Questions

He was placed in a specially prepared bed.
Was he placed in a specially prepared bed?

She was given a suitable premedication.
Was she given a suitable premedication?

1 He was given an intramuscular injection.
2 They were asked to sign a consent form.
3 They were allowed frequent sips of water.
4 Her leg was put in plaster of Paris.
5 They were told to come back tomorrow.
6 These instruments were sterilized.
7 The patient was placed on his back.
8 The injections were given at 6 o'clock.

The Past Perfect Tense

Active			*Passive*		
I		gone	I		told
You		heard	You		asked
He		assisted	He		taken
She	had	seen	She	had been	seen
It		come	It		used
We		helped	We		shown
They		asked	They		sent

The past perfect tense is used for an action in the past which happened before another action, also in the past, for example

The doctor *told* them that John *had sustained* a fracture.

The nurse *took* John's pulse and blood pressure after she *had admitted* him.

Soon after John *had returned* to the ward, he began to regain consciousness.

The past perfect is often used with

before, after, as soon as, until, when

E

Complete the following sentences with the past perfect tense

1 We (give) .... him first aid by the time the ambulance arrived.

2 The doctor wanted to know what the nurse (do) ....

3 Mary didn't get home until after her parents (go) .... to bed.

4 I found my way to the clinic after I (ask) .... the theatre sister the way.

5 You lost your new gloves soon after you (buy) .... them, didn't you?

6 When John (recover) .... from his operation, he was sent home.

7 The doctor did not arrive until the patients (finish) .... their breakfast.

8 As soon as the surgeon (examine) .... the x-rays, he started the operation.

F

Complete the following sentences with the correct past simple or past perfect tense of the verb in brackets

Remember, the past perfect marks the *earlier* of the actions.

1 The nurse who admitted John (ask) .... what (happen) .... to him.

2 He (tell) .... her that he (be knocked) .... down.

3 Mary (work) .... at the hospital for six months before she (meet) .... Jane.

4 When the nurse (set) .... the trolley, she (take) .... it into the ward.

5 After the disposable instruments (be used) .... they (be thrown) .... away.

6 After the surgeon (examine) .... the patient, he (tell) .... him there was nothing to worry about.

7 Jane's headache (not, get) .... better until she (take) .... several Aspirins.

8 The radiographer (tell) .... the patient not to move until she (take) .... the x-ray.

9 When she (take) .... the x-rays, the radiographer (take) .... the patient back to the ward.

10 After they (have) .... their dinner, they (go) .... to the cinema.

11 The surgeon who (perform) .... the operation (visit) .... John next morning.

11 — The Ward Unit 1

The ward is the patient's home during his stay in hospital. It is the place in which he spends his days, eats and sleeps, and where his personal needs are catered for. A well-planned ward provides a pleasant, safe and comfortable environment for patients and staff.

The planning of ward units for new hospitals, and for modernization schemes in older ones, has received a great deal of consideration. In the past, in-patients were allowed up only for short periods during convalescence. The modern practice of early ambulation has made it essential to provide adequate space for recreation and sufficient bathing and toilet facilities. Bright colours have been used to create a cheerful atmosphere in the ward, and furniture has been designed to suit the different needs of patients.

Another problem on which hospital planners have focused their attention is the reduction of unnecessary noise. The use of plastic equipment, and the provision of central dish-washing and sterilizing departments have been a great help in eliminating noise.

The question of ward cleaning has also been taken into consideration by the planners. Nowadays the floors and walls are made of materials that can withstand very frequent washing and polishing. Furniture and fittings have been designed to permit easy cleaning and maintenance.

A

Answer the following questions

1 What does the patient do in the ward?

2 What is done for the patient in the ward?

3 Name three things that have received attention in the planning of new hospitals.

4 Where did in-patients spend most of their time in the past?

5 When were in-patients allowed up in the past?
6 What is the modern practice?
7 What facilities has this modern practice made essential?
8 How have planners reduced noise in modern hospitals?
9 What are the floors and walls made of nowadays?
10 How have new furniture and fittings been designed?

B

Vocabulary

We can say

1 The ward is the place where the patient's needs are taken care of.
or
It's the place where the patient's needs are ....

2 Ward planning has received much thought.
or
Ward planning has received ....

3 A patient who is kept in hospital
or
An ....

4 Patients were allowed up for short periods while they were getting better.
or
They were allowed up for short periods ....

5 The modern practice of getting patients walking as soon as possible
or
The modern practice of ....

6 There is sufficient space.
or
There is .... space.

7 Bright colours are used to produce a cheerful atmosphere.
or
Bright colours are used .... a cheerful atmosphere.

8 Planners have concentrated their attention on noise problems.

or

They have .... their attention on noise problems.

9 This has been a great help in getting rid of noise.

or

This has been a great help in .... noise.

10 The question of maintenance has been considered by the planners.

or

The question of maintenance ....

.... by the planners.

11 Something has been designed to allow easy cleaning.

or

Something has been designed .... easy cleaning.

12 The setting up of central dish-washing departments has been a great help in eliminating noise.

or

The .... central dish-washing departments has been a great help in eliminating noise.

C

Complete the following sentences with the correct prepositions

1 The ward is the patient's home .... his stay .... hospital.

2 It is the place .... which he spends his days and where his needs are catered ....

3 A well-planned ward provides a comfortable environment .... both patients and staff.

4 The planning .... new ward units has received a great deal .... attention.

5 In–patients spent most of their time .... bed .... the past.

6 Early ambulation has made it essential to provide adequate space .... recreation.

7 A problem .... which hospital planners have focused their attention is the reduction .... unnecessary noise.

8 The use .... plastic equipment and the provision .... central dish–washing departments have been a great help .... eliminating noise.

The Present Perfect Tense

Active

<table>
<tr><td>I
You
We
They</td><td>have</td><td rowspan="2">gone
asked
recovered
helped
seen
taken
eliminated</td></tr>
<tr><td>He
She
It</td><td>has</td></tr>
</table>

Passive

<table>
<tr><td>I
You
We
They</td><td>have</td><td rowspan="2">been</td><td rowspan="2">injured
told
hurt
examined
x-rayed
prepared
sterilized</td></tr>
<tr><td>He
She
It</td><td>has</td></tr>
</table>

The present perfect is used for actions and states in the past when no definite time is mentioned. The actions could have taken place at any time in the past up to the present. It is often used with *just, yet, already, never* and *since.*

I have just seen the nursing officer.
Jane has already finished her work.
Mary has never been in hospital before.
Jane has not qualified yet: she is still a student nurse.

D

Complete the following sentences with the correct form of the present perfect tense of the verbs in brackets

1 The doctor .... just (speak) .... to the sister.

2 She (not, ask) .... for the patients' notes yet.

3 He (be) .... in this ward for the last three weeks.

4 Early ambulation (make) .... it essential to provide a lot of space.

5 Jane's bus .... already (go) ....

6 Hospital planners (focus) .... their attention on noise problems.

7 Colour-schemes and the design of furniture (receive) .... a great deal of attention.

8 These patients ...... never (have) .... operations before.

Compare the following sentences:

I have seen him before.
I saw him last Saturday.
We haven't finished the course yet.
We finished the course yesterday.
Have they seen her?
Did they see her last night?

The present perfect is used when no definite time is mentioned. The past simple is used when a definite time is mentioned.

E

Complete the following sentences with the correct tense, either present perfect or past simple

1 Doctors (use) .... disinfectants for nearly one century.

2 Scientists (discover) .... many new antibiotics since the last war.

3 Sir Alexander Fleming (discover) .... penicillin in 1928.

4 Since the 1930's, the search for better antibiotics (continue) ....

5 Lord Lister (use) .... carbolic acid to prevent infection at the end of the last century.

6 Nurse Smith (work) .... at St. Peter's since she (qualify) .... in 1967.

7 Joan (take) .... the patient to the x-ray department yesterday.

8 Nurse Smith (just, take) .... a patient to theatre.

Drill 1 Present perfect – questions

You have hurt your leg.	*Have you hurt your leg?*
He has had his operation.	*Has he had his operation?*

1 She has seen the sister.
2 They have studied physiology.
3 The instruments have been sterilized.
4 The patient has been catheterized.
5 You have visited the gynaecological ward.
6 We have seen the operating theatre.
7 Ward planning has received attention.
8 He has found her notes.

Drill 2 Present perfect – negatives

He has broken his leg. *He hasn't broken his leg.*

She has seen the nursing officer. *She hasn't seen the matron.*

1 It has been sterilized.
2 I have seen Dr Wilson.
3 She has prepared the trolley.
4 The patient has arrived.
5 They have come to see her.
6 His leg has been fractured.
7 This patient has been catheterized.
8 He has had an injection of morphine.

Drill 3

Use the diagram to practise asking the way using sentences such as
Could you show me the way to the sluice, please?

Would you mind showing me the way to the sluice, please?

Diagram of a Typical Ward

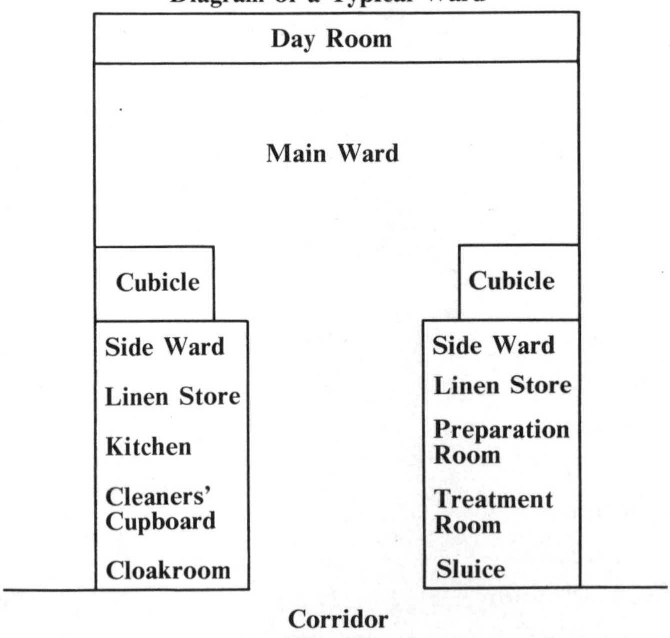

12 — The Ward Unit 2

Accommodation for patients

Most modern hospital wards have between twenty and thirty beds. The beds are arranged so that each patient can have as much privacy, natural light and fresh air as possible, and can be observed without difficulty by the nursing staff. There must be adequate space between beds to prevent cross-infection and to allow all bedside procedures to be carried out in comfort.

Most wards have a number of cubicles or side wards – usually six for a thirty-bed ward – and two of these have their own hand basins and lavatories so that suitable accommodation is available for infectious patients. Ambulant patients and patients in wheelchairs are provided with a day room where they can have their meals, watch television, smoke and enjoy various recreations without disturbing patients who are confined to bed.

Lavatories and bathrooms are sufficiently spacious to allow nurses to assist old and disabled patients. Doorways are wide enough to allow wheelchair patients to enter with ease. The rooms are usually fitted with grab-rails, shelves and hooks, and a patient-to-nurse alarm system is provided. It is important that lavatories flush quietly and efficiently.

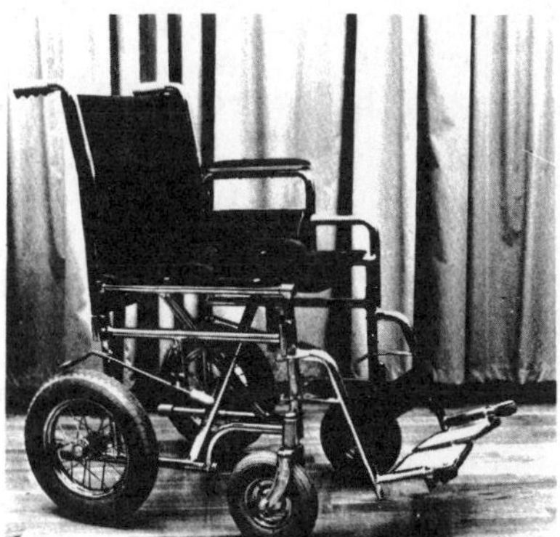

wheelchair

A

Answer the following questions

1 How many beds have most modern hospital wards?
2 How many cubicles or side wards are there?
3 What have two of these cubicles or side wards usually got?
4 Where are infectious patients accommodated?
5 Why must there be adequate space between beds in the ward?
6 For whom is the day room provided?
7 What do these patients do in the day room?
8 Why must lavatories and bathrooms be sufficiently spacious?

B

Read the text carefully and complete the following sentences

Do not look back at the text until you have tried to do all the sentences.

In modern hospital wards, patients' beds are arranged so that each patient has as much p................, n................... light and f.......... a........ as possible. There must be a.................... space between beds to prevent c........-...................... Most wards have a number of c................. or s........ wards so that there is suitable a....................... for i....................... patients.

A day room is provided for a................... patients and patients in w...................... In the day room, they can enjoy various r....................... without disturbing patients who are c....... .... t.... b.......... Lavatories and bathrooms must be large enough to allow nurses to assist old and d................ patients. These rooms are usually fitted with g.......-..........., hooks and shelves, and a patient-to-nurse a.............. system is provided.

C

Complete the following sentences with the correct form of the verbs in brackets

1 In the past hospital wards (have) .... very many beds.

2 The ward where I work (have) .... 16 beds.

3 Nurse Smith (start) .... working here in 1967.

4 The gynaecological consultant usually (do) .... a round at 10 a.m. on Tuesdays.

5 I saw Jane while I (wait) .... for the bus.

6 These instruments (sterilize) .... yesterday.

7 Three new patients (admit) .... yesterday.

8 The nurse who admitted the new patient (give) .... him an anti-tetanus injection.

9 While the patient (wait) .... to go to theatre, a quarter-hourly record of his blood pressure was kept.

10 He (give) .... a suitable premedication one hour before he was taken to theatre.

D

Rewrite the following pairs of sentences as one sentence using 'who' or 'that' when necessary

1 The patient is John's father. You were talking to him yesterday.
2 The instruments are sterile. They are in this box.
3 Antiseptics are chemical substances. They inhibit the growth of micro-organisms.
4 Someone phoned for an ambulance. He saw the accident.
5 The book is very interesting. I am reading it.
6 The patient is going home now. You admitted him last Thursday.

7 The doctor told his parents an operation was necessary. The doctor had examined John.

8 The doctor is the orthopaedic consultant. John's parents spoke to him.

E

Ask the patient

1 when the accident happened.
2 if he has had pneumonia before.
3 who her general practitioner is.
4 if he has been immunized against tetanus.
5 if he has been in hospital before.
6 if his leg hurts.
7 when he woke up this morning.
8 if she slept well last night.
9 if he is feeling better.
10 if there is anything you can get for him.
11 if he would like to sit in the day room.
12 where the pain is.
13 if he has had the same pain before.
14 when the pain started.
15 if he has taken his medicine.

F

What do the following abbreviations stand for?

1 S.R.N.
2 C.S.S.D.
3 t.p.r.
4 a.m.
5 p.m.
6 E.N.T.
7 Mgs.

G

What instrument do you use

1 to remove stitches?
2 to handle sterile instruments?
3 to remove Michel's clips?
4 to give an injection?
5 to explore a wound?

13 — The Ward Unit 3

Clinical areas

In the treatment room of a ward unit, surgical dressings, investigations and other sterile procedures can be carried out under optimal conditions and with minimal risk of cross-infection. The treatment room should be large enough to accommodate a patient in his bed, a couch for ambulant patients, and all the equipment needed for treatments. It must of course allow medical and nursing staff adequate space to work in comfort.

Next to the treatment room, there are usually a 'clean' and 'dirty' annex. The clean annex, or preparation room, is where trolleys are laid up. If there is no C.S.S.D., equipment and instruments are sterilized there too. The preparation room is provided with dust-proof cupboards in which sterile equipment is stored. In the dirty annex, used equipment is collected and cleaned, or kept for collection by the C.S.S.D.

Near the dirty annex, there is usually a sluice room. The sluice room has facilities for cleaning and sterilizing bedpans, urinals, sputum mugs and so-on, and for disinfecting soiled bed linen. In many wards, one corner of the sluice room is provided with a bench, sink and the necessary equipment for testing urine. The arranging of flowers is also normally done in the 'sluice'.

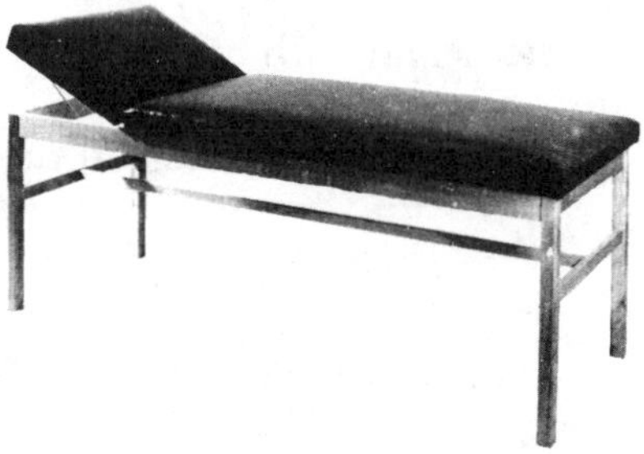

examination couch

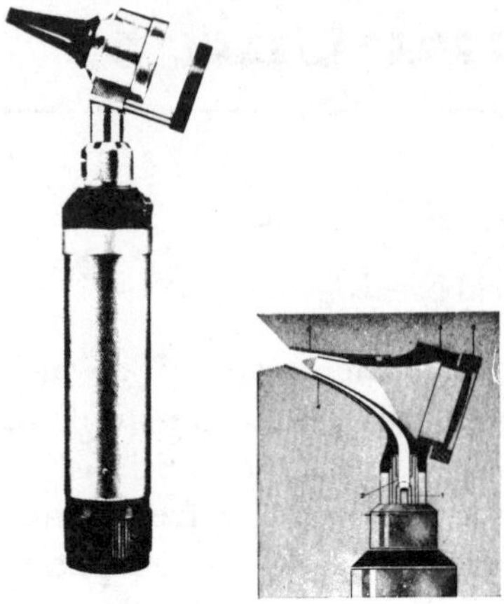

auriscope

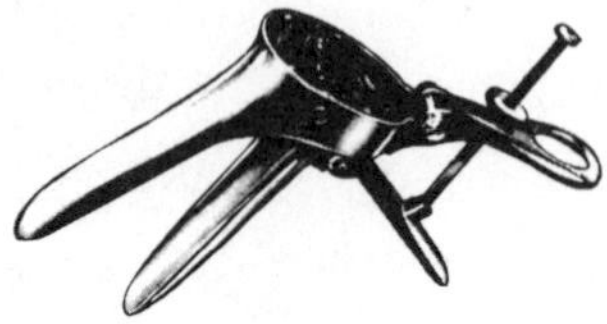

vaginal speculum

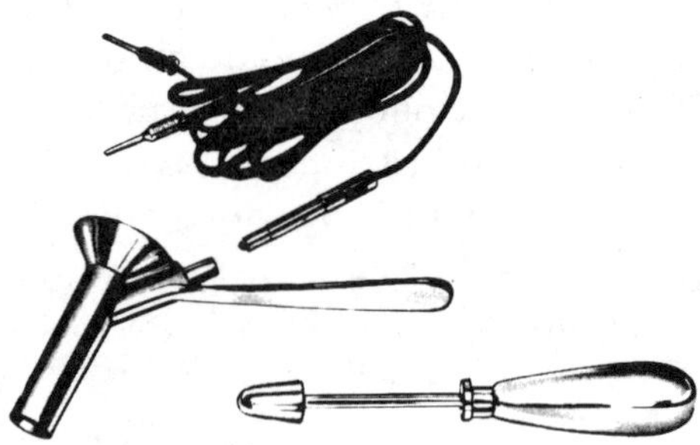

proctoscope, or rectal speculum

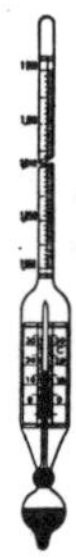

urinometer

A

Read the text carefully and complete the following sentences

In the treatment room various surgical procedures are carried out under

o.................. conditions and with m................ risk of

c........–.................... The treatment room is big enough to hold

a patient in his bed, a c.......... for a.................. patients, and

all the e...................... needed for treatments. It is also large enough

to allow medical and nursing staff a................. space to work in comfort.

Next to the treatment room, there are usually a 'clean' and a 'dirty' a........

The clean a............ or p.................... room is where trolleys are laid up and if there is no C.S.S.D., equipment and i.............. are sterilized there too. It is provided with d.......-.......... cupboards in which sterile equipment can be stored. In the dirty annex, soiled equipment is collected and cleaned, or kept for collection by the C................

Next to the dirty annex there is often a s.................. room. It has f................. for cleaning and s..................... bedpans, u................. and s............ mugs. It also has f............ for d.................... soiled bed l............. In one corner of the sluice room there is often a b................, a s............ and the necessary equipment for testing u.............

B

Complete the following sentences with the correct prepositions

1 A day room is provided ....ambulant patients and patients in wheelchairs.

2 Bathrooms and lavatories are provided .... hooks and shelves.

3 There is a couch .... ambulant patients in the treatment room.

4 Adequate space between beds in the ward helps to reduce the risk ...... cross-infection.

5 There are facilities .... sterilizing bedpans in the sluice.

6 The arranging .... flowers is usually done in the sluice.

Purpose

Look at these sentences

The beds are arranged *so that* patients can have as much fresh air as possible.

There must be adequate space between beds *to prevent* cross-infection.

Furniture and fittings have been designed *to permit* easy cleaning.

John's leg was x-rayed *so that* the surgeon could see the exact site and extent of the fracture.

C

Complete the following sentences with 'so that' or a suitable infinitive with 'to'

1 A day room is provided .... ambulant patients have somewhere to relax.

2 The patient was given an antibiotic .... the onset of infection.

3 The doorways are always wide enough .... patients in wheelchairs to enter with ease.

4 Some side wards have their own basins and lavatories .... suitable accommodation is provided for infectious patients.

5 The beds are arranged .... patients can be observed without difficulty.

6 Hospital planners have used bright colours .... a cheerful atmosphere.

7 The patient was given an injection of morphine .... shock and pain.

8 Jane studied hard .... she could pass her examinations.

9 Furniture and fittings are designed .... they can be cleaned easily.

10 Mary made notes at the lecture .... she could remember the important points.

Question-tags

With a positive statement, we have a negative tag

She is a gynaecologist, isn't she?
You have seen the treatment room, haven't you?
He likes ice-cream, doesn't he?
She will come, won't she?
They often visit him, don't they?

With a negative statement, we have a positive tag

She isn't a gynaecologist, is she?
You haven't seen the treatment room, have you?
He doesn't like ice-cream, does he?
She won't come, will she?
They don't visit him often, do they?

D

Supply the missing question tags

1 The syringe is sterile, ...?

2 He has had his injection, ...?

3 He's not a consultant, ...?

4 They are radiographers, ...?

5 You're not going, ...?

6 They did it, ...?

7 This is the dispensary, ...?

8 This isn't the preparation room, ...?

9 They weren't staff nurses, ...?

10 John was admitted yesterday, ...?

11 She went home last week, ...?

12 You will help me, ...?

13 It won't hurt, ...?

14 It doesn't hurt, ...?

15 There are enough beds, ...?

16 She can walk, ...?

17 It wasn't difficult to find, ...?

18 You found them, ...?

19 He will get better, ...?

20 This equipment isn't sterile, ...?

21 You have given her a bedpan, ...?

22 She is on duty, ...?

23 Nurse Brown admitted him, ...?

24 You will come tomorrow, ...?

Drill

Supply question tags and try to make your voice rise and fall correctly

Statement This isn't disinfectant.

With tag This isn't disinfectant, is it?

Now go on

1 This isn't disinfectant.
2 The treatment room wasn't large.
3 The sluice should be tiled.
4 Ward flowers can be attractive.
5 Contaminated bed linen must be destroyed.
6 The doctor can scrub up here.
7 Doorways ought to be wide.
8 Supper isn't ready yet.

14 — The Ward Unit 4

The sister's office

A sister's office, usually situated near the ward entrance, is provided for general administration. In the office, medical and nursing staff can have privacy to discuss the treatment and progress of patients. The sister's office is also used by medical-social workers and the hospital chaplain for interviewing patients and relatives.

Domestic and storage areas

The domestic and storage areas of a ward include the kitchen, the linen and equipment store, the cleaners' room and the staff cloakroom. The kitchen has facilities for making hot drinks and preparing light meals, and for washing up. The linen and equipment store is used for storing blankets, sheets and pillow-cases, and bulky equipment such as bed cradles, portable backrests and cot sides. If the linen store is sufficiently spacious, stretchers and wheelchairs are often 'parked' there. The cleaners' room is usually near the ward entrance, and is used for storing brooms, buckets, mops, vacuum cleaners and cleaning materials. The staff cloakroom is also usually near the entrance of the ward. It has wash-basins and lavatories, personal lockers and facilities for hanging clothes.

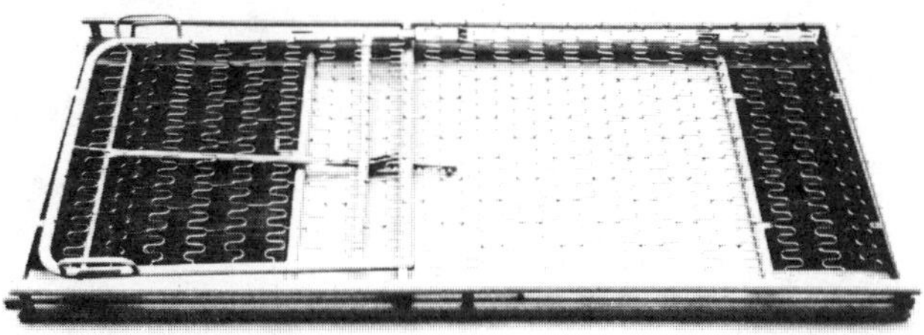

portable backrest

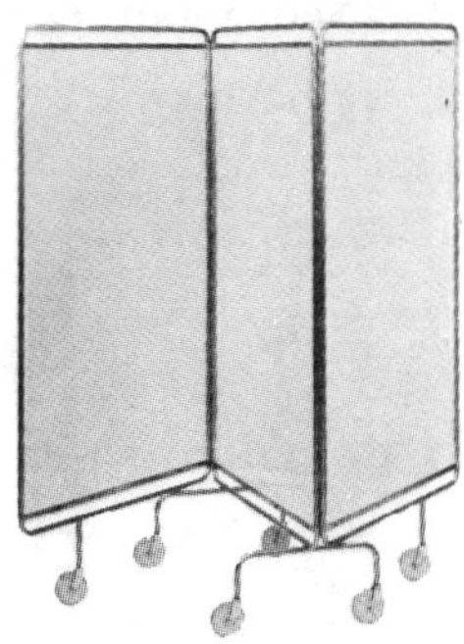

screens

A

Answer the following questions

1 Where is the sister's office situated?
2 Who uses the sister's office?
3 Where are patients and their relatives interviewed?
4 What facilities has the ward kitchen?
5 Where is bed linen kept?
6 Where is bulky equipment stored?
7 What are often parked in the linen store?
8 Where would you look for cleaning materials?
9 Where is the staff cloakroom often situated?
10 What facilities has the staff cloakroom?

B

In what hospital ward or department would you expect to find

1 a patient who has had his appendix removed?
2 a patient who has had his tonsils out?
3 a patient with a broken leg?
4 someone who has just had an accident?
5 a patient with cerebral haemorrhage?
6 an elderly patient?
7 someone who is having an operation?
8 a patient with a skin disease?
9 a woman who will have a baby in two months' time?
10 a patient who is being admitted?
11 a radiographer?
12 a pharmacist?

C

In which part of the ward unit

1 do patients relax, smoke and watch TV?
2 are infectious patients nursed?
3 can surgical procedures be carried out under optimal conditions?
4 is used equipment collected and cleaned?

5 are trolleys prepared?
6 are bedpans, urinals etc. sterilized?
7 is urine tested?
8 is sterile equipment stored?

Plans with 'going to'

The Hospital Secretary is talking to a visiting Member of Parliament about plans for the future

"We're going to build a new ward unit this year. The builders are going to start in March. The new unit is going to have thirty beds. There will be six side wards with their own lavatories, a modern treatment room, a preparation room, and a sluice room – for disinfecting equipment, routine urine testing and so on. The ward sister's office is going to be very nice: it'll be near the entrance so that patients won't be disturbed. We're going to use bright colours everywhere and, of course, low-maintenance furniture and fittings. The scheme is going to cost £250,000. ... Now I'm going to take you to lunch."

We usually use *going to* . . . when talking, informally, about plans or events in the near future.

D

Complete the following sentences with 'going to'

1 I (have) .... a holiday next month.

2 Joan (meet) .... her friend this evening.

3 Mr and Mrs Smith (visit) .... John in hospital tomorrow.

4 She (marry) .... an engineer.

5 Now I (examine) .... you, so please take off your shirt.

6 Who (choose) .... the colours for the new ward unit?

Not going to

Look at these sentences. Notice where we put 'not' or 'n't'.

I'm not going to be at home next month.
Joan isn't going to study this evening.
We aren't going to operate on that patient.

Drill

Supply question tags

1 You haven't any privacy in this ward.
2 They'll be discharged on Monday.
3 You didn't feel that.
4 We could understand the tutor.
5 We mustn't be late.
6 She oughtn't to lay up like that.
7 He needs a bed-cradle.
8 You won't be late.
9 He does work hard.
10 You have confidence in the surgeon.
11 He can come on Thursday.
12 She ought to be ashamed.
13 We needn't work late.
14 We must get a new urinometer.

OFFASON AB, OXIE 1974

15 — Admissions

In Britain, most people who fall ill are treated at home by their family doctors. Not all illnesses can be treated at home, however, so many people are admitted to hospital at some time during their lives. They are admitted either as arranged admissions or as emergency admissions.

Arranged Admissions

A patient who goes into hospital as an arranged admission has previously attended an out-patients' clinic to which he has been sent by his family doctor. At the clinic he is examined, his previous history is taken and all the necessary investigations are carried out. If admission is recommended, his name is put on a waiting list and when a bed in an appropriate ward becomes vacant, he is sent a letter which tells him when to report to the hospital for admission. With this letter, most hospitals enclose a leaflet telling the patient what he will need while he is in hospital. The leaflet also outlines the general ward routine and gives details of visiting hours.

Emergency Admissions

Nowadays, many people go into hospital as a result of accidents or sudden illnesses. These patients are called emergency admissions. They are often seriously ill and in need of immediate care and attention. Unlike arranged admissions, little or nothing is known about emergency admissions or their previous histories. They are usually taken to the casualty and emergency department by ambulance. They are often unconscious. Sometimes they are accompanied by friends or relatives who are able to supply at least their personal particulars. In the casualty department, they are examined and the necessary emergency treatment is carried out. If possible their previous histories are taken. The appropriate ward is notified that a patient is being sent up so that the necessary preparations can be made.

A

Read through the text and answer the following questions with complete sentences

1 Why are most people admitted to hospital at some time during their lives?
2 What sort of clinic has an arranged admission previously attended?
3 What is done if admission is recommended?
4 What is the patient sent by the hospital?
5 What does the leaflet sent by the hospital tell the patient?
6 Why are patients admitted as emergencies?
7 What is known about emergency admissions?
8 What information can the friends and relatives of emergency admissions give us?
9 What happens to an emergency admission in the casualty department?
10 Why is the ward notified that a patient is being sent up?

B

Vocabulary

What words in the text mean the same as

1 someone who comes to hospital as a result of a sudden illness or accident

....

2 to tell someone you have arrived .... someone

3 facts about a person's health in the past ....

(medical) ....

4 facts about a person's age, sex, height, weight, married-or-single, etc.

....

5 following, or because of ....

6 not knowing — feeling — seeing, etc., anything at all

....

7 proper, suitable, correct ....

8 a printed sheet of paper giving information about a certain subject

....

C

Complete the following sentences by supplying the correct form of the verb

1 He (be) ill with pneumonia since June.
2 I (have) a pain before I came to the clinic but it (go) now.
3 When the telephone rang, I (do) the t.p.rs.
4 While sister (phone) for the doctor I (give) mouth-to-mouth resuscitation.
5 Dead tissue (remove) by the surgeon.
6 The patient (tell) the police that he (hit) by a car an hour ago.
7 He (give) a pre-med ten minutes ago.
8 His headache (not, get) better until he (take) an Aspirin.
9 He (come) to work when he had a heart attack.
10 These patients (catheterize) last night.

16 — Arranged Admission

A patient who has been on the waiting list for admission has received a letter telling him to report to Dixon ward at Cambury Hospital for admission on 24th July at 2.30 p.m. At 2.30 he arrives at the sister's office.

Here is the admission card she filled in:

CAMBURY HOSPITAL Admission Card	Hosp. Reg. No. Ward/Dept.
SURNAME (IN BLOCK LETTERS) MC LEOD	FIRST NAME(S) PETER JOHN
ADDRESS & TELEPHONE NO. 26 GREENEND, WATERBEACH WATERBEACH 234	DATE OF BIRTH 21. 12. 1934
CIVIL STATE Married ~~Single~~ ~~Widowed~~ ~~Other~~	OCCUPATION (In the case of a child, father's occupation.) CARPENTER
RELIGION C. of E.	NAME & ADDRESS OF NEXT OF KIN MARY MCLEOD (wife) As above
NAME & ADDRESS OF G.P. DR BEALE THE OAKS, HIGH ST., LANDBEACH	TELEPHONE NO. (If not on the phone, give a number where messages may be sent. Add 'Messages only'.)
SURGEON OR PHYSICIAN IN CHARGE OF CASE MR THORPE	

Here is what they said

Patient	Excuse me, nurse. Is this Dixon ward?
Sister	Yes, this is Dixon.
Patient	Well, I'm Peter McLeod. You sent me a letter telling me to report here at half past two.
Sister	That's right, Mr McLeod. Would you come in and sit down, please? We have to fill in an admission card.
Patient	Thank you.
Sister	Now, your surname is McLeod—would you mind spelling it, please?
Patient	M C capital L E O D.
Sister	Thank you. And your Christian names?
Patient	Peter John.
Sister	Where do you live?
Patient	26 Greenend, Waterbeach.
Sister	Are you on the phone?
Patient	Yes. Waterbeach 234.
Sister	And when were you born?
Patient	21st December 1934.
Sister	Are you married?
Patient	Yes, I am.
Sister	And what's your occupation?
Patient	I'm a carpenter.
Sister	What's your religion?
Patient	Church of England.
Sister	It says here, 'Name and address of next of kin'. Who is your nearest relation?
Patient	My wife, Mary.
Sister	And you live at the same address?
Patient	Yes, of course.
Sister	Now, who is your family doctor?
Patient	Dr Beale.
Sister	And his address?

Patient	The Oaks, High Street, Landbeach.
Sister	Do you know which doctor is in charge of your case?
Patient	Er... I believe it's Dr Thorpe.
Sister	Ah yes. Mr Thorpe—he's a surgeon, you see. Well, thank you, Mr McLeod. If you would just wait here for a few minutes, I'll get a nurse to come and take care of you.

A

Practise these questions

Where do you live?
What's your religion?
Who's your nearest relation?
(And) what's your occupation?
(And) when were you born?
(Now,) who's your family doctor?

Are you married?
Are you on the phone?
Do you know which doctor is in charge of your case?

(And) your Christian names?
(And) his address?
(And) you live at the same address?

Would you sit down, please?
Would you mind spelling it, please?

B

Interview your neighbour

Ask the type of question the sister used in the dialogue and fill in this form.

Surname	....
First Names	....
Address	....
Phone Number	....
Date of Birth	....
Civil State	....
Religion	....
Occupation	....
Next of Kin	....

Would you mind spelling it, please?

This form of request is usually considered polite enough without 'please'. Remember 'Would you mind' is followed by the -ing form.

C

Make the following polite requests

1 open the window
2 close the door
3 spell your name
4 repeat the question
5 notify the ward
6 ring casualty
7 fill in this form
8 help me with this
9 give her a cigarette
10 take him to x-ray

D

Supply question tags to the following sentences

1 You haven't been in hospital before, . . . ?
2 You were born on 28th February 1936, . . . ?
3 Your religion is Church of England, . . . ?
4 That's not your office telephone number, . . . ?
5 Your parents are still alive, . . . ?
6 You've brought some pyjamas, . . . ?
7 You didn't bring any medicines with you, . . . ?
8 You've had a cold recently, . . . ?
9 Your wife will be visiting you tonight, . . . ?
10 You can remember the way to the toilet, . . . ?

E

Vocabulary

Fill in the blanks

The sister wrote down the patient's p. . . . . p. . . . . on an a. . . . . c. . . . . She wrote in b. . . . . l. . . . . She knew his surname but asked him what his C. . . . . n. . . . . .s were. She wrote 'CARPENTER' under O. . . . . and crossed out all the words except 'Married' under C. . . . . S. . . . . The patient said his N. . . . . . . o. . . K. . . . . . . was his wife and his D. . . . . o. . . B. . . . . was 21-12-1934.

The sister noted that Mr Thorpe was i. . . c. . . . . o. . . the case.

17 — Observation of the Patient

After admission, general observation of the patient is made regularly. Here the staff nurse is telling the student about observing patients.

Staff You know that we have to keep an eye on all patients all the time, don't you?

Student Yes, we have to keep on the look out for changes in their condition.

Staff That's right. What sort of changes?

Student Er, changes in t.p.r., changes in colour. What mental state he's in. And of course anything on his record card. I must say it seems an awful lot. How do we find the time to do it?

Staff You must get into the habit of observing the patients when you're carrying out normal nursing duties. After a time it becomes second nature.

Student They gave us a list of things to look for in training school. I expect I'll get used to it soon.

Staff Don't forget that it's very important to chat to patients. If you get on friendly terms with them it's a great help.

Student Why?

Staff Well it makes them more relaxed. Also they may tell you something about their lives which has some bearing on their illness.

Student And what about the quiet ones?

Staff There may be a lot of reasons why they don't want to talk to you. They may be frightened. They may be depressed. They may not be able to speak the language. The important thing is that even though you're rushed off your feet you must find time to talk to people. You'll be surprised how important it is.

A

Answer the following questions

1 Who has to observe the patients in a ward?
2 What do they have to look for?
3 What may a change in a patient's temperature indicate?
4 Do you only have to observe the patient's physical state?
5 When do you observe patients?
6 Should the nurses keep themselves to themselves?
7 Why do you think that it is important to have patients who are relaxed?
8 Why may some patients be reluctant to talk to you?
9 Should you talk to patients if you are busy?
10 Who are the people on the ward who come into most contact with the patients?

B

Vocabulary

Give words or phrases that mean the opposite of

Example hot: *cold*

1 to have one's bowels open: to be c ....

2 depressed: e...................

3 anxious: c ....

4 rushed off one's feet: r ....

5 encouraging: d................ing.

C

Fill in the blanks

We can say

1 watch carefully or o.........................., or k.............

an.........................

2 way of acting or b.......................

3 precisely or a...........................

4 state or c.....................

5 tell one's troubles to or c............... in.

6 shy and withdrawn or r......................

7 unhelpful or un.......................

8 tell or n..............y, or i................m.

9 empty, free or v....................t.

10 wound or i.........................y.

18 — The Skin

The skin is the outer covering of the body. It consists of two coats: the epidermis or cuticle, and the dermis or corium. Beneath these, there is a layer of adipose tissue which connects the skin to the underlying structures. This layer is known as the subcutaneous layer.

Diagram of a section of the skin

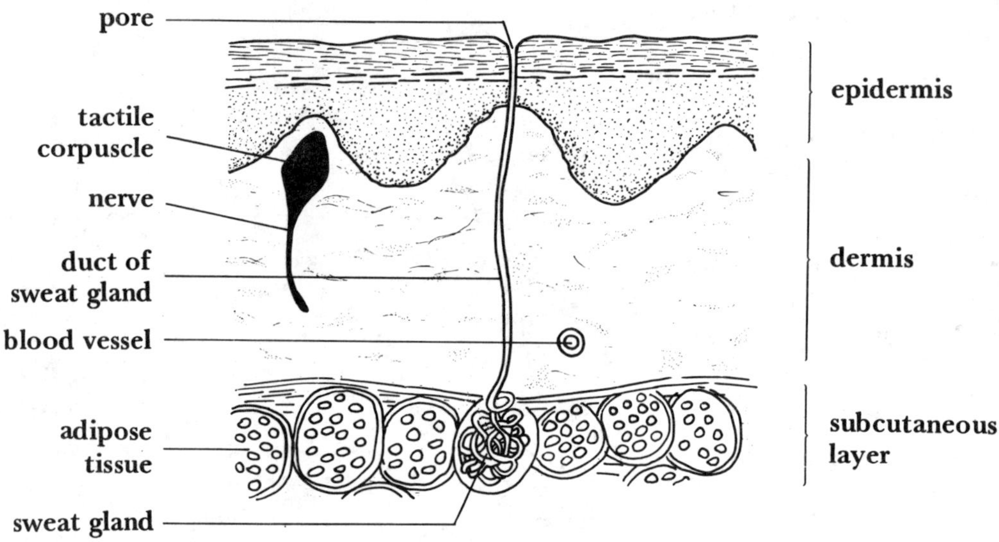

The skin is usually warm, dry and elastic, but changes in its condition can occur both in illness and in health. The skin of patients who are dehydrated as a result of prolonged pyrexia is dry and inelastic. In some infectious diseases, it is hot and wet due to hyperpyrexia and profuse sweating. In cases of shock and haemorrhage, it is cold and clammy. In skin diseases, it can be either excessively moist or excessively dry and scaly.

The colour of the skin can also vary considerably. It can be flushed in pyrexia, pallid in shock, cyanosed in anoxaemia or yellowish in jaundice.

A

Answer the following questions with complete sentences

1 Which two layers does the skin consist of?
2 Which layer connects the skin to the underlying structures?
3 What is the normal condition of the skin?
4 What is the condition of the skin in dehydrated patients?
5 What can cause dehydration?
6 When can the skin be hot and wet?
7 When is the skin cold and clammy?
8 When can the skin be excessively dry and scaly?
9 What colour can the skin be in patients with fever?
10 What is the colour of the skin in patients suffering from shock?
11 What is the colour of the skin in patients who have too little oxygen in their blood?
12 What colour is the skin in jaundiced patients?

B

Medical terms often seem long and unnecessarily complicated. However, if we stop to study them a little more closely, we shall see that they are by no means as difficult as they first appeared. They are usually made up of simpler parts which we have taken from Greek or Latin. Let us examine some of the words derived from Greek and Latin that we have in this lesson.

Dermis	Pyrexia
Epidermis	Hyperpyrexia
Cuticle	Haemorrhage
Subcutaneous	Pallid
Corpuscle	Cyanosed
	Anoxaemia

C

Vocabulary

Make a list of new words in the text

Divide them up into columns

Names for parts of the skin	Conditions, Diseases and Symptoms	Adjectives and Adverbs
epidermis	*pyrexia*	*dehydrated*
....	....	....
....	....	....
....	....	....
....	....	....
....	....	....
....	....	....
....	....	....
....	....	....
....	....	....
....	....	....
....	....	....
....	....	....
....	....	....
....	....	....
....	....	....

What words are left?—What do they mean?

D

Label the diagram

Try not to look at the labelled diagram on the first page of this lesson until you have finished. Another way to practise is to give the numbers and ask a friend to give the names.

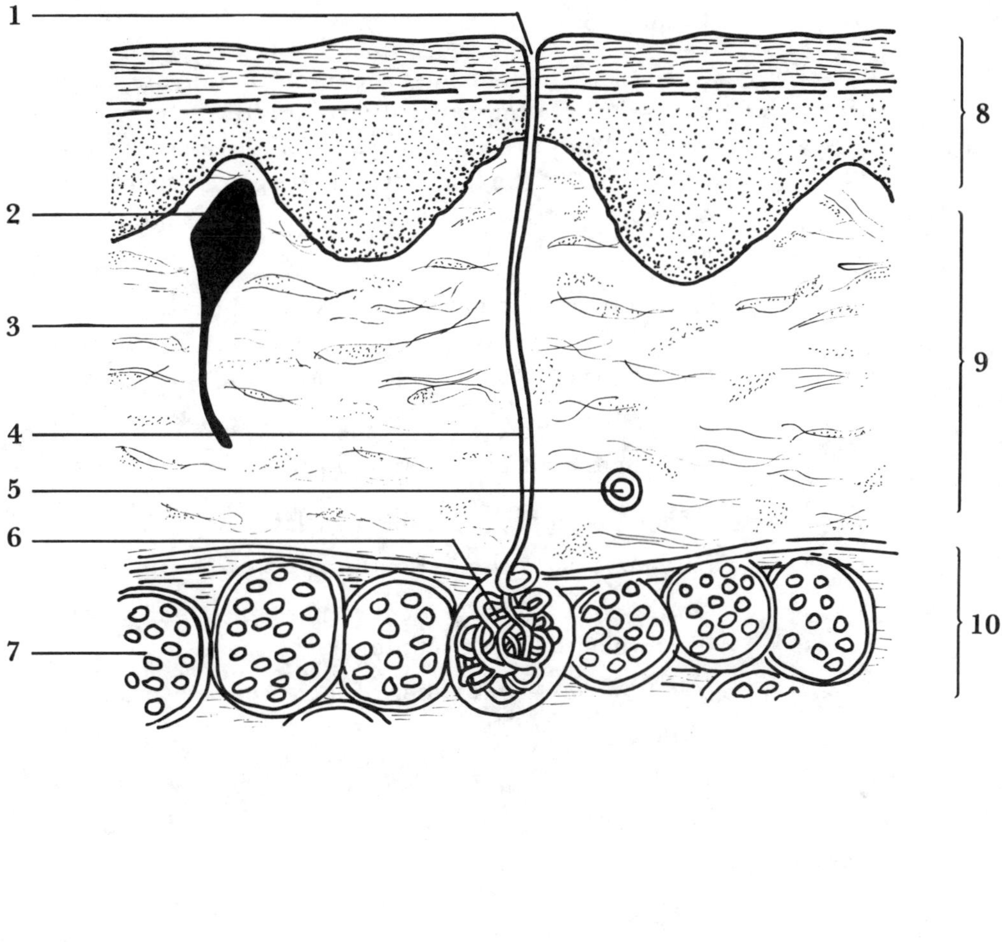

19 — Respiration, the Cough and Sputum

Respiration

Changes in the rate and type of respiration are one of the principal symptoms of disorders of the respiratory system. They are also symptoms of diseases affecting other parts of the body. Respiratory disturbances can be seen in cardiac disease, cerebral depression, uraemia and diabetic coma.

When observing a patient, the rate and depth, and the ease or difficulty of breathing are noted. It is also important to observe whether breathing is noisy or quiet.

The following are some of the terms commonly used to describe the different types of respiration:

Apnoea – a period during which breathing is absent

Dyspnoea – difficult breathing

Orthopnoea – the patient can breathe comfortably only when sitting or standing erect

Hyperpnoea – breathing of increased rate and depth

Shallow breathing – seen when chest movements are painful

Stertorous breathing – noisy, snoring breathing

The cough

Coughing is a reflex action which occurs when the respiratory passages are irritated. Coughing expels irritants such as excess sputum and foreign bodies from the respiratory tract. A cough is known as non-productive when no sputum is expectorated, and when sputum is expectorated, the cough is known as productive.

Sputum

The following terms are used to describe various types of sputum:

Mucoid sputum is clear, tenacious mucus which is produced in the early stages of respiratory tract infection.

Mucopurulent sputum is a mixture of mucus and pus which is produced in the later stages of respiratory tract infection.

Purulent sputum consists mainly of pus, and is seen in cases of bronchiectasis and lung abscess.

Rust-coloured sputum is tenacious and contains altered blood. It occurs in cases of lobar pneumonia.

Haemoptysis is the term used to describe the coughing up of bright red, frothy blood from the lungs. It is seen in cases of pulmonary tuberculosis, carcinoma of the lung and bronchiectasis.

Diagram of the respiratory system

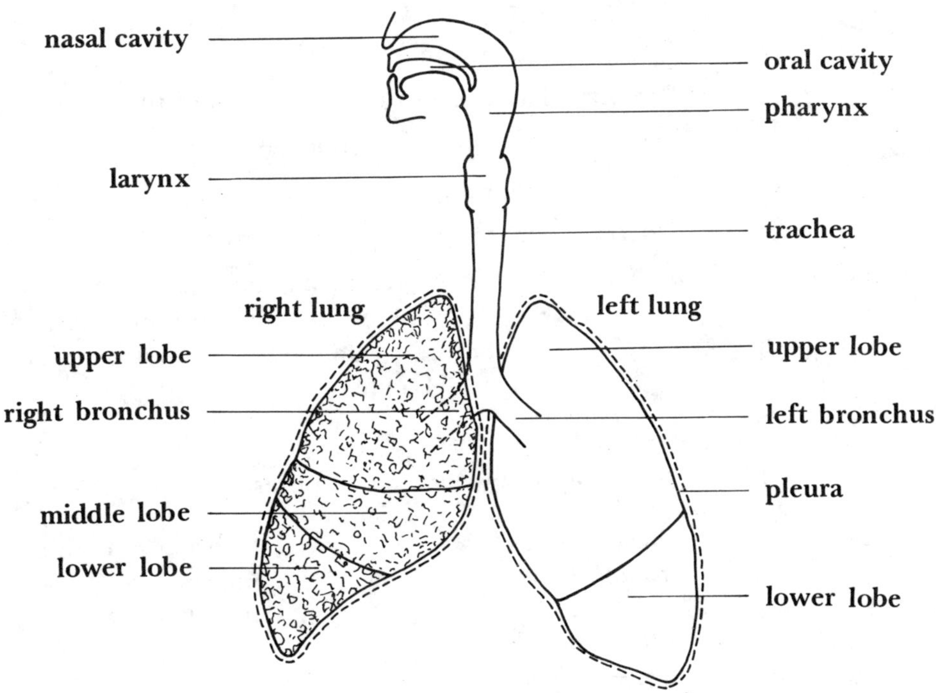

Interview

A patient with chest trouble and a high temperature has come to the casualty and emergency department of a hospital. Here is part of the interview between the patient and a doctor

Doctor	Good afternoon, Mrs Williams. I'm Doctor Martin. Now, you're having some trouble with your chest, aren't you?
Patient	Yes, doctor, I am. I've got a terrible cough and a pain down here in my chest.
Doctor	How long have you had the cough?
Patient	Oh, it started about a month ago . . . a nasty tight cough . . . then it seemed to go away. Then, about a week ago, it came back again.
Doctor	Are you bringing anything up when you cough?
Patient	Yes. The last couple of days I've been bringing up sticky, reddish-brown phlegm.
Doctor	Next time you bring something up, I'd like you to spit it into this mug, please.
Patient	O.K.
Doctor	Do you smoke much?
Patient	No . . . not really. Fifteen to twenty a day.
Doctor	Have you ever coughed up any blood?
Patient	No, never.
Doctor	Have you had a temperature?
Patient	Well, I've been feeling feverish for two or three days. I took my temperature this morning . . . just before I came here . . . and it was 102. Oh, I feel awful!

Some important words and phrases

chest trouble
trouble with one's chest
a tight cough
a loose cough
nasty

to bring something up
phlegm
to cough up
feverish

A
Practise these sentences

Are you having chest trouble?
Are you having trouble with your chest?
Is it a tight cough?
Is it a loose cough?
Are you bringing anything up when you cough?
Do you smoke much?
Have you ever coughed up any blood?
Have you had a temperature?

I'm having chest trouble.
I'm having trouble with my chest.
I've got a terrible cough.
I've got a nasty, tight cough.
I've got a loose cough.
I've been bringing up sticky, reddish-brown phlegm.
I'd like you to spit it into this mug, please.
I've been feeling feverish for two or three days.
I took my temperature this morning.
I feel awful!

B
Vocabulary

1	We can say	main or most important or p ....
2	Another word for	disease, condition, something wrong is d ....
3	We can say	cough up or ex ....
4	Instead of saying	distance from top to bottom, we can say d.......................................
5	We can say	standing or sitting or pointing up or ....

6 Another word for throw out is e..............................

7 Another word for too much is e..............................

8 Instead of saying an unwanted substance or object, we can say

a f............... b ....

9 Instead of saying holding on, adhesive, sticky, we can say

t..................................

10 We can say a collection of pus somewhere in the body or

an ....

11 We can say made up of many small bubbles or

f..................................

12 Instead of saying of the lungs, we can say p ....

C

Complete the following sentences

1 Sputum consisting of mucus and pus is known as ....

.... sputum.

2 Breathing of increased rate and depth is known as h................

3 A tight cough is one that produces no sputum: it is also known as a

.... cough.

4 Absence of breathing is known as ....

5 .... is the term used to describe the coughing up of blood from the lungs.

6 .... breathing is noisy, snoring breathing.

7 A productive cough is one which produces sputum: it is also known as a

l.............. cough.

8 Sputum consisting mainly of pus is known as .... sputum.

9 .... breathing is the type of breathing seen when chest movements are painful.

10 Sputum seen in pneumonia is often ....-coloured.

11 .... is the term used to describe a condition in which the patient can breathe with comfort only when he is sitting or standing erect.

12 .... sputum is clear, tenacious mucus.

D

Label this diagram

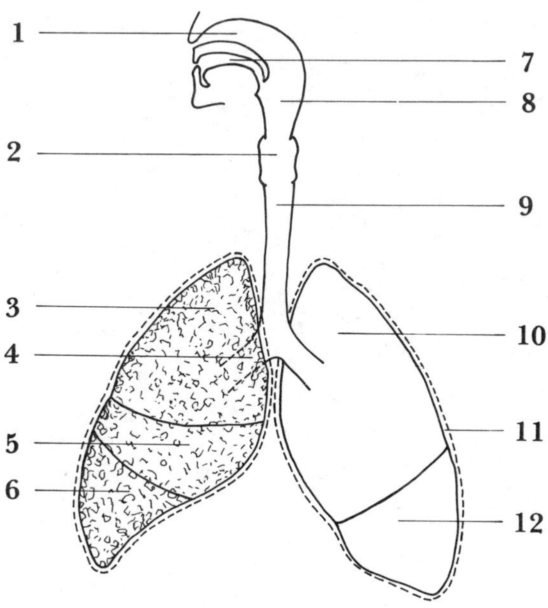

20 — Vomitus

When a patient is sick, the contents of the stomach are ejected through the mouth. These ejected stomach contents are correctly known as vomitus. Vomitus usually consists of partially-digested food, but may consist of bile, blood or a foul-smelling, brown fluid. Vomiting, or emesis, is one of the principal symptoms of disorders of the digestive system but it is also a symptom of many other illnesses.

When vomiting is a symptom, the consistency of the vomitus and the frequency of vomiting are noted. The patient is asked whether nausea precedes vomiting, if pain is present and whether it is relieved by vomiting. It is also important to ascertain whether vomiting occurs in connection with the taking of food and, if it does, whether it occurs immediately after or some time after a meal.

Diagram of the digestive system and associated glands

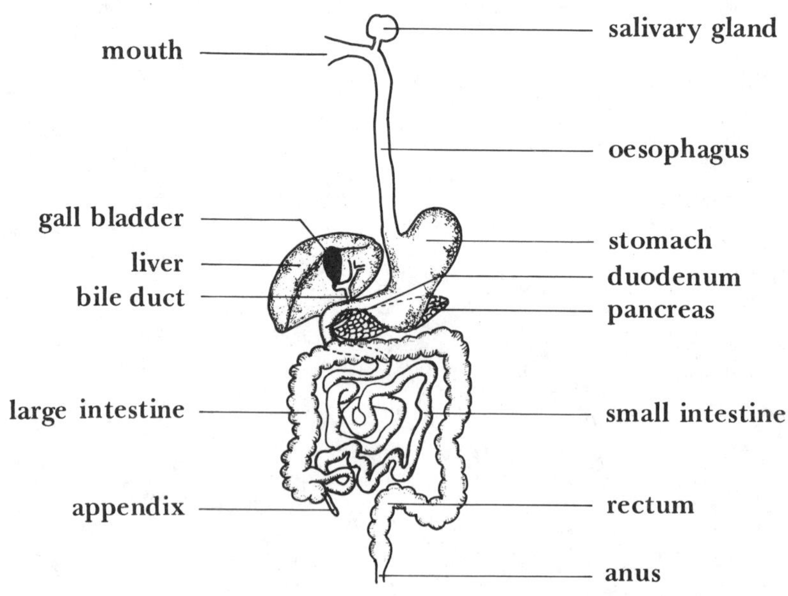

A nurse who is taking t.p.rs has a chat with Mr Smith

Patient Hello, nurse.

Nurse Hello, Mr Smith, how are you feeling this morning?

Patient Not too bad, thanks, but I am feeling a bit queasy.

Nurse Have you been sick?

Patient Not this morning, but I was sick as a dog just after you went off duty yesterday afternoon.

Nurse Oh? After you'd had your tea?

Patient No. Before tea. All of a sudden I was violently sick.

Nurse Did you have nausea before you were sick?

Patient Pardon?

Nurse Did you feel queasy before you were sick?

Patient No. It came on suddenly.

Nurse Did you have any pain?

Patient No. None at all. I was feeling fine. Then I was sick. Then I felt fine again.

Nurse But you're feeling a bit queasy now?

Patient Well, I'm not really sure, perhaps I'm imagining it.

Nurse It's nothing to worry about. We'll tell Dr Higgins when he does his round and see what he says.

Patient I suppose it could have been the chocolates.

Nurse Chocolates?

Patient Well, I had visitors yesterday afternoon, you know. They brought me a box of Black Magic. I was a bit lonely when my visitors went . . . there's one chocolate left . . . would you like it?

Important words and phrases

not too bad, thanks.	all of a sudden
queasy	to come on
to be sick	to go off
as sick as a dog	pardon?

A

Practise these sentences

How are you feeling this morning?

Not too bad, thanks.

I'm feeling a bit queasy.

Have you been sick?

I was sick as a dog yesterday afternoon.

All of a sudden I was violently sick.

Did you have nausea before you were sick?

Did you feel queasy before you were sick?

Pardon?

It came on suddenly.

It went off suddenly.

Did you have any pain?

No. None at all.

Perhaps I'm imagining it.

It's nothing to worry about.

We'll tell Dr Higgins when he does his round.

We'll see what he says.

B

Answer the following questions with complete sentences

1 What are ejected through the mouth when a patient is sick?
2 What are the ejected contents of the stomach correctly known as?
3 What does vomitus usually consist of?
4 What may vomitus consist of?
5 What is vomiting one of the principal symptoms of?
6 What details are noted when a patient is sick?
7 What is the patient asked?
8 What is it also important to ascertain?

C

Label the diagram

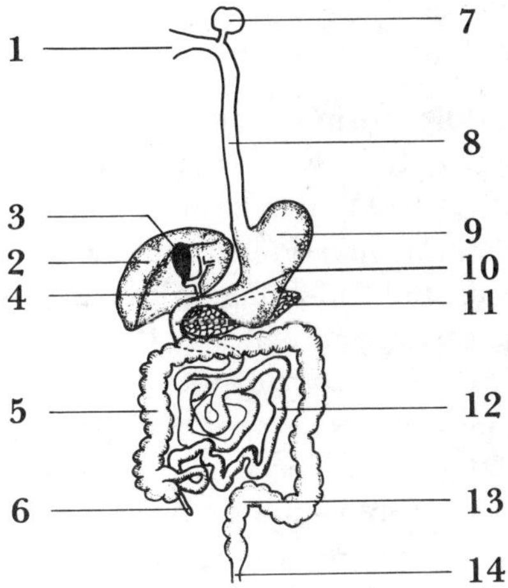

D

Vocabulary

1 We can say vomiting or ....

2 Bones are solid, flatus is a gas and blood is f.........................

3 Another word for thickness, firmness of a substance is c.............

4 We can say feel sick or have n.................

5 Instead of saying come before, happen before, we can say p..........

6 We can say help, lighten or ....

7 We can say find out or a....................

8 Instead of saying together with, we can say in c............... with.

9 We can say it started suddenly or it .... suddenly.

10 We can say it stopped or it ....

11 We can say the secretion of the liver or b..........

21 — Faeces

In the adult, normal faeces are brown, semi-solid and have a characteristic odour. Faeces consist of indigestible or undigested food, altered bile pigments, water, mucus, cells from the intestinal tract, and bacteria. When observing faeces, the following points are noted: the frequency of defaecation and whether flatus is passed, the colour and consistency of the stools, and the presence of any abnormal substances or objects. Fresh blood in a stool is usually due to bleeding in the lower bowel. Altered blood in a stool is due to bleeding in the stomach or small intestine and produces dark, tarry stool—melaena. The absence of bile pigments and the presence of large amounts of fat produce stools that are putty-coloured and extremely offensive.

Constipation is a condition in which the passing of stools is difficult and infrequent.

Diarrhoea is a condition in which frequent loose or liquid stools are passed.

Stomach trouble

Mr Mills has a history of stomach trouble. He has an appointment at a medical out-patients' clinic at 14.30 on Monday, July 1st. He arrives on time, and after a few minutes, the doctor is ready to see him.

Doctor Good afternoon. Mr Mills, isn't it?

Patient Yes. Good afternoon, doctor.

Doctor Sit down, please. Now, let me see, you've been having trouble with your stomach, haven't you?

Patient Yes. I have this pain, and now my stools are all black and tarry.

Doctor How long have you had the pain?

Patient Oh, for about two years. But it's been getting much worse since the beginning of May.

Doctor	Do you have it all the time?
Patient	No, it comes on about an hour to an hour and a half after I've had a meal.
Doctor	Does it last long?
Patient	No. I usually have a biscuit and a glass of milk, and then it goes off.
Doctor	Have you ever vomited any blood?
Patient	Never.
Doctor	Have you been feeling weak or tired or cold?
Patient	Well, I have been feeling a bit weak since I came home from my holidays.
Doctor	When was that?
Patient	Three weeks ago.
Doctor	For how long have you been passing these tarry stools?
Patient	Since last Friday.
Doctor	Are they loose?
Patient	No, they're not. They're all black and hard.
Doctor	How often do you have your bowels open?
Patient	Once a day. I usually take a laxative.
Doctor	Well, thank you, Mr Mills. Now would you mind undressing? I'd like to examine you.

A

Practise these sentences

Now, let me see.
You've been having trouble with your stomach, haven't you?
My stools are all black and tarry.
How long have you had the pain?
For about two years.
It's been getting much worse since the beginning of May.
Do you have it all the time?
No, it comes on after I've had a meal.
Does it last long?
I usually have a glass of milk and then it goes off.

Have you ever vomited any blood?

For how long have you been passing these tarry stools?

Since last Friday.

Have you been feeling weak?

I've been feeling a bit weak since I came home from my holidays.

When was that?

Three weeks ago.

Are your stools loose?

How often do you have your bowels open?

I usually take a laxative.

Would you mind undressing?

Since – For

Look at these sentences

It's been getting much worse since *the beginning of May.*
I've been feeling a bit weak since *I came home from my holidays.*
I've been passing these tarry stools since *last Friday.*

I've had the pain for *about two years.*
She's been waiting for *three hours.*
He's been in hospital for *months.*

We use *since* when a *definite point in time* is mentioned.
We use *for* when a *length of time* is mentioned.

B

Look at these examples

He began studying orthopaedics in 1962.
He's been studying orthopaedics since 1962.

She started working at the hospital last Monday.
She's been working at the hospital since last Monday.

Now you change the sentences in the same way

1 It started hurting in the middle of January.
2 He started coughing up blood last June.
3 I started passing tarry stools on Wednesday.
4 The gynaecologist started operating at 10.30.
5 She began smoking heavily at Christmas.
6 He began vomiting blood this morning.
7 The pain started getting worse last Easter.

C

Look at these examples

She began waiting three hours ago.
She's been waiting for three hours.

I began feeling ill a month ago.
I've been feeling ill for a month.

Now you change the sentences in the same way

1 It started hurting about three weeks ago.
2 He began complaining about the pain a year ago.
3 I started attending the out-patients clinic two months ago.
4 I began bringing up phlegm two days ago.
5 He started feeling weak a fortnight ago.
6 It began raining half an hour ago.
7 She started taking laxatives six months ago.
8 They started living in Sweden years ago.

D

Complete the following sentences with since or for

1 I've coughed up blood several times .... I last saw the doctor.
2 I've been waiting to see the physiotherapist .... half an hour.
3 He hasn't had any trouble with his chest .... 1967.
4 Have you passed any tarry stools .... you last saw me?

5 She's been having stomach trouble .... months.

6 He's been in theatre .... an hour.

7 They've been waiting to see him .... 9.30.

8 He's been complaining of pain .... the last three weeks.

9 I've had trouble with my breathing .... I had pneumonia.

10 He's had heart trouble .... years.

E

Vocabulary

Complete the following sentences

1 If something cannot be digested, it can be called ....

2 If something has not been digested, it is ....

3 We can say, the passing of faeces, or ....

4 We can talk about gas or air in the bowels or ....

5 We can say, altered blood in the stool, or ....

6 We can say, organic colouring matter, or ....

7 We can say, the intestines, or the ....

8 We can say, an unpleasant smell, or an unpleasant ....

9 If someone passes frequent, loose stools, he has ....

10 If someone passes stools with difficulty and irregularly, he has

....

11 We can ask, how often do you pass faeces? or ....

....

12 We can say, a medicine which helps defaecation, or a ....

22 — Urine

Normal urine is an amber fluid which consists of approximately 96 % water, 2 % urea and 2 % salts. It has a slightly acid reaction, and a specific gravity of between 1·004 and 1·025. The amount of urine passed depends on the fluid intake and the needs of the body. When the fluid intake is decreased, or when there is profuse sweating, excessive emesis or diarrhoea, the volume of urine passed is decreased. It is darker and has a higher specific gravity than usual.

When the fluid intake is increased, and in cold weather, the volume of urine passed is increased. It is lighter and has a lower specific gravity than usual.

Diagram of the urinary system

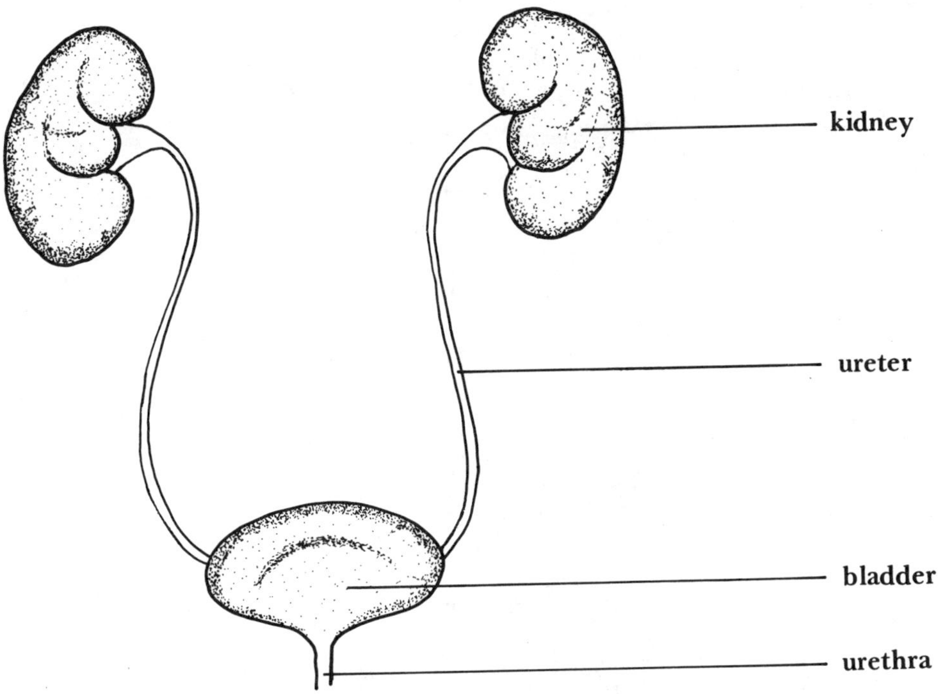

The following terms are used to describe abnormalities in the excretion of urine:

Polyuria – an increase in the amount of urine excreted.

Oliguria – a decrease in the amount of urine excreted.

Dysuria – difficult micturition.

Anuria or suppression – failure of the kidneys to excrete urine.

Retention – urine is excreted by the kidneys but retained in the bladder.

Frequency – micturition occurs more frequently than usual.

Incontinence – absence of control over the passing of urine.

Haematuria – the presence of blood in the urine.

Proteinuria or albuminuria – the presence of protein in the urine.

A

Answer the following questions

1 What is the medical term for difficulty in passing water?
2 What is another way of saying anuria?
3 What four things can lead to oliguria?
4 What is the opposite of acid?
5 What can cause urine to have a higher specific gravity than usual?
6 When is urine darker than usual?
7 What is a commoner way of saying to micturate?
8 What is the medical term for absence of control of micturition?
9 How is the production of urine affected by cold weather?
10 What is another way of saying haematuria?

B

Label this diagram

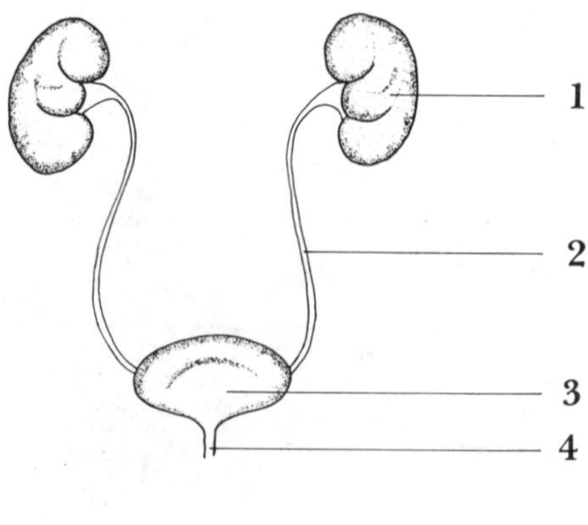

Fluid balance chart

NAME	AGE	WARD	HOSPITAL REG.NO.

24 HOUR INTAKE IN Mls.					24 HOUR OUTPUT IN Mls.			
Date	Oral	I.V.	Other Routes	Total	Urine	Vomit or Aspiration	Drainage	Total

23 — Temperature

Human beings maintain an almost constant body temperature. The normal temperature of some adults is as low as 97 °F and in others, it is as high as 99 °F. There is also a normal daily variation of about one degree. The temperature is lowest in the early hours of the morning and highest in the evening.

Body heat is produced by metabolic and muscular activity. It is lost by evaporation of sweat from the skin, expiration of air from the lungs and excretion of urine and faeces.

The balance between heat production and heat loss is maintained by the heat-regulating centre in the hypothalamus, which is sensitive to minute variations in the temperature of the blood passing through it.

A rise in blood temperature produces an increase in the flow of blood to the surface of the body. Sweat gland activity is increased, muscle tone is diminished and there is unwillingness to move about.

A fall in blood temperature produces a decreased flow of blood to the superficial vessels. There is decreased activity of the sweat glands, increased muscle tone and a desire to move about. Shivering, which is a reflex contraction of the muscles, may occur to increase heat production.

Fahrenheit and Centigrade

The Fahrenheit thermometric scale extends from 0° to 212°. 0 °F = −18 °C, 32 °F = 0 °C (freezing-point) and 212 °F = 100 °C (boiling-point). Normal body temperature is 98·4 °F.

To convert degrees Fahrenheit into degrees Centigrade, we subtract 32, multiply by 5, and divide by 9.

Example 100 °F

$100 - 32 = 68$

$68 \times 5 = 340$

$340 \div 9 = 37 \cdot 7$

$\therefore$ 100 °F = 37·7 °C

To convert from Centigrade into Fahrenheit, we multiply by 9, divide by 5, and add 32.

Example 25 °C

$25 \times 9 = 225$

$225 \div 5 = 45$

$45 + 32 = 77$

$\therefore$ 25 °C = 77 °F

A

Which words in the text have the same meaning as

1 near the surface ....

2 unchanging ....

3 alteration ....

4 extremely small ....

5 decreased ....

6 breathing out ....

7 controlling ....

8 changing into vapour ....

9 reluctance ....

10 discharge of waste products ....

B

Write five sentences using the following verbs

1 to maintain
2 to produce
3 to increase
4 to decrease
5 to occur

T.P.R. CHART

Name | Hosp no.

First names | Date of Birth | Sex

Consultant | Ward

MONTH

DAY

		M. E. (×21 days)	
TEMPERATURE	41		105·8
	40		104
	39		102·2
	38		100·4
	37		98·6
	36		96·8
PULSE	150		150
	140		140
	130		130
	120		120
	110		110
	100		100
	90		90
	80		80
	70		70
RESPIRATION	60		60
	50		50
	40		40
	30		30
	20		20
	10		10
BLOOD PRESSURE			BLOOD PRESSURE
FLUID INTAKE			FLUID INTAKE
URINE	Volume		Volume
	Specific Gravity		Specific Gravity
	Reaction		Reaction
	Albumin		Albumin
	Sugar		Sugar
VOMIT			VOMIT
BOWELS			BOWELS

24 — Pulse

The pulse is the wave of distension produced in the arteries when the left ventricle of the heart contracts and pumps blood into the aorta. It is most easily felt where a large superficial artery crosses a bone. The most convenient point is on the anterior surface of the wrist, where the radial artery crosses the radius.

The pulse rate is the frequency of the heart beat. This can vary considerably. The normal pulse rate of some adults is as slow as 50 per minute, and others as fast as 90 per minute: the average is said to be 72. In the infant, the pulse rate can be as rapid as 140.

The pulse volume indicates the amount of blood in circulation, and the propulsive power of the heart.

The pulse rhythm is normally even in time and force, but irregularities occur in health and in illness. In all cases where irregularities are noted, the heart apex beat is counted. The apex beat can be located in the fifth intercostal space about two inches to the left of the sternum.

Diagram of the thoracic cage

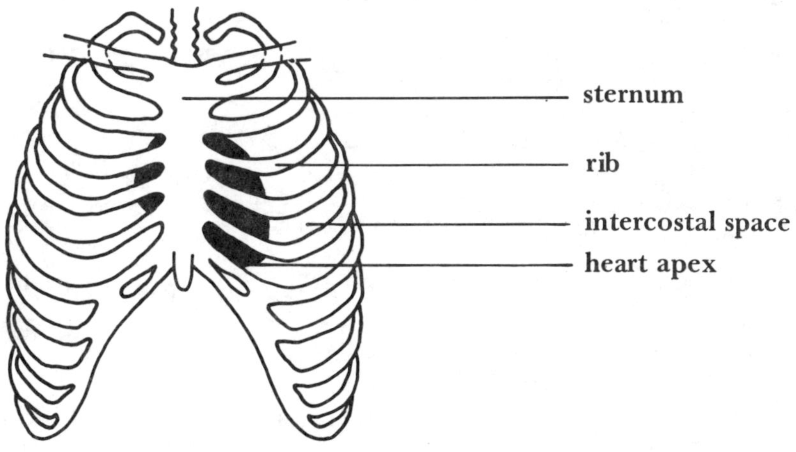

Comparison of adjectives

Look at these sentences

Pulse rate is not normally *slower than* 50 per minute.
This patient's temperature is *as high as* it was yesterday.
Temperature is *lowest* in the morning and *highest* in the evening.
The patient's temperature was *the highest* we have ever recorded.

With long adjectives, we usually use *more/less* and *most/least*:

The most convenient point to take a person's pulse is on the anterior surface of the wrist: it is *less convenient* to take the apex beat.

A

Fill in the missing words

1 Normal urine is (light) .... urine passed when the fluid intake is decreased.

2 The patient is feeling (good) .... she was yesterday.

3 He received (expensive) .... treatment available.

4 Pulse rate is usually (high) .... after exercise.

5 The pain is (bad) .... it was yesterday.

6 This is (bad) .... attack of asthma I've ever had.

7 It was (large) .... cyst the surgeon had ever removed!

8 Mr Smith was (sick) .... a dog this morning.

9 She's (uncooperative) .... patient in the ward!

10 The new chemical thermometers are (convenient) .... mercury thermometers.

Comparison of adverbs

Look at these sentences

Pulse rate is *most easily* felt at the wrist.
She recovered *more quickly than* they had expected.
His temperature decreased *less rapidly than* they had hoped.

We usually use more/less and most/least for short adverbs as well as for long ones.

B

Fill in the missing words

1 You will get home (quick) .... by taxi .... on foot.

2 Autoclaving sterilizes (efficient) .... boiling.

3 Rabbits are (high) ....-developed .... humans, but some people say they are .... fertile.

4 Good, his heart is beating (strong) .... it was an hour ago.

5 I'm glad to say she comes for check-ups (regular) .... she used to.

When?

Prepositions of time

We say *at* for *fixed points of time*	at half past three
We say *on* for *days of the week*	I have my hair done on Mondays.
We say *in* for *periods of time*	in summer, in February, in 1969, in the morning

C

Fill in the blanks with at, on or in

1 ...... Mondays, I go on duty ...... six o'clock ...... the morning and come off duty ...... two o'clock ...... the afternoon.

2 He never works ...... night.

3 She was born ...... 1928.

4 My birthday is ...... January.

5 I have holidays ...... Christmas, ... Easter and ...... the summer.

6 What shall we do ...... Sunday?

7 Where were you ...... Thursday evening?

8 ...... the evenings, we watch 'the box'.

9 The patient woke up several times .... night.

10 Our club usually meets ...... the second Thursday ...... the month, but ...... the summer, we meet ...... the weekend instead.

D

Label this diagram

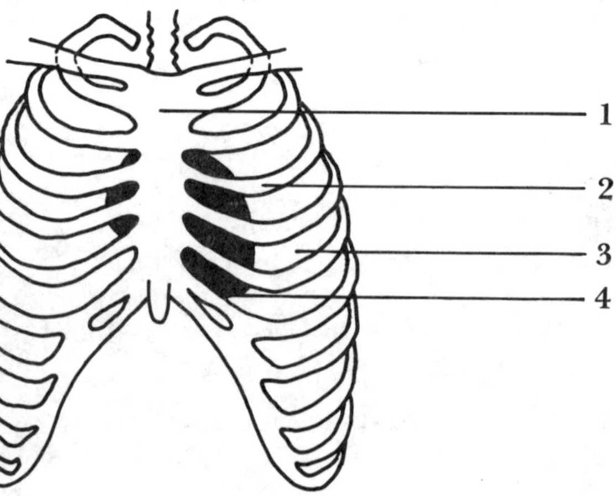

E

Expressions of time in relation to 'now'

This table is for you to write phrases like "yesterday, three days ago, in three weeks' time" and so on. Your teacher will help you to build up the table.

			today			
			this week			
			this month			
			this year			
			this season			
			this spring			
			this summer			
			this autumn			
			this winter			
			this term			

F

Vocabulary

1 Instead of saying the left ventricle gets smaller, we can say the left ventricle c................ .

2 Blood flows from the heart through the ....ies.

3 Blood returns to the heart through the ....s.

4 Instead of talking about the blood's journey round the body, we can say the c..................... of the blood.

5 The top, or sharpest, point of a triangle is its ....

6 Instead of saying a pulse, we can say a w........... of d.............

7 Another way of saying increase in size is d.....................n.

8 Instead of saying can be found, we can say can be ....

9 One word for between the ribs is ....

10 The ribs are attached to the s............... anteriorly.

(A..................... is another word for in front.)

11 Another word for to show is to ....

12 We can say pushing power or p.................... power.

Word List

This list contains technical medical words that occur in the book, as well as many of the non-technical words that are needed in running a hospital. The pronunciation of each word is shown, followed by the number of the unit where the word is first used. (Note that a few words, especially names of drugs, may be used in exercises without occurring in the reading passages or dialogues.)

Meanings are given. Many medical terms have similar forms in most languages, and the meaning of others will often be clear from the passage where they occur. In cases of doubt, the following dictionaries may be useful:

Nancy Roper, *Livingstone's Pocket Medical Dictionary*

William A. R. Thomson, *Thomson's Concise Medical Dictionary*

Both are published by Churchill Livingstone.

Pronunciations are shown in the system that is used in the new *Dictionary of Contemporary English* (Longman). The symbols are shown in this table, with a key word for each; the letters printed in **bold type** represent the sound value of the symbol.

Consonants

p	**p**ea	f	**f**ew	ʃ	fi**sh**ing	h	**h**ot
b	**b**ay	v	**v**iew	ʒ	plea**s**ure	m	su**m**
t	**t**ea	θ	**th**ing	tʃ	**ch**oose	n	su**n**
d	**d**ay	ð	**th**en	dʒ	**j**ump	ŋ	su**ng**
k	**k**ey	s	**s**oon	l	**l**ed	j	**y**et
g	**g**ay	z	**z**oo	r	**r**ed	w	**w**et

Vowels

iː	sh**ee**p	ɔː	c**augh**t	eɪ	m**a**ke	ɪə	h**ere**
ɪ	sh**i**p	ʊ	p**u**t	əʊ	n**o**te	eə	th**ere**
e	b**e**d	uː	b**oo**t	aɪ	b**i**te	ʊə	p**oor**
æ	b**a**d	ʌ	c**u**t	aʊ	n**ow**	eɪə	pl**ayer**
ɑː	c**al**m	ɜː	b**ir**d	ɔɪ	b**oy**	əʊə	l**ower**
ɒ	c**o**t	ə	cupb**oar**d			aɪə	t**ire**
						aʊə	t**ower**
						ɔɪə	empl**oyer**

Notes

1 A small raised [^{r}] at the end of a word means that the [^{r}] is pronounced if a vowel follows (at the beginning of the next word), but not otherwise. For example, *far* [fɑː^{r}] means that *far away* is pronounced [ˌfɑːr əˈweɪ] but *far down* would be [ˌfɑː ˈdaʊn].

2 The italic [*ə*] means that the sound [ə] can be used but is usually omitted. It will be found before the consonants [m, n, ŋ, l, r]. For example, *travel* [ˈtræv*ə*l] means that the pronunciation [ˈtrævəl] is possible but [ˈtrævl] is normal and should be used if possible.

3 The mark ['] means that the following syllable has *main stress*, and [ˌ] means that the following syllable has *secondary stress*—for example, *understand* [ˌʌndə'stænd].

4 The following abbreviations are used to indicate parts of speech where pronunciation differs according to the part of speech:
n noun; *v* verb; *adj* adjective; *adv* adverb

abscess ['æbses] (19) a collection of pus
adipose ['ædɪpəʊz] (18) fat
administer [əd'mɪnɪstəʳ] (4) to give
airway ['eəweɪ] (9) trachea or instrument for ventilation
albumen ['ælbju:mɪn] a variety of protein
albuminuria [ælˌbju:mɪ'njʊərɪə] (22) albumen in the urine
ambulant ['æmbjʊlənt] (12) able to walk
anaesthetic [ˌænəs'θetɪk] (12) a drug which produces lack of feeling
anatomy [ə'nætəmɪ] (3) science of the structure of the body
anoxaemia ['ænɒk'si:mɪə] (18) no oxygen in the blood
antenatal [ˌæntɪ'neɪtl] (1) before birth
anterior [æn'tɪərɪəʳ] (2) in front of
anti- ['æntɪ] (8) against
antibiotic [ˌæntɪbaɪ'ɒtɪk] (9) a drug which destroys bacteria
antiseptic [ˌæntɪ'septɪk] (5) substances which destroy or make difficult the growth of germs
anuria [æ'njʊərɪə] (22) lack of urine
anus ['eɪnəs] (20) end of the digestive system
aorta [eɪ'ɔ:tə]. (24) main artery coming from the left ventricle of the heart
apex ['eɪpeks] (24) the beat of the heart
apnoea [æp'nɪə] (19) temporary stop to breathing
appendix [ə'pendɪks] (20) small blind tube coming from the large intestine—it has no known function.
artery ['ɑ:tərɪ] (6) vessel carrying blood away from the heart
aspiration [ˌæspɪ'reɪʃən] (22) the act of breathing in
Aspirin ['æsprɪn] (10) mild pain killing drug
asthma ['æsmə] (24) a sudden attack of difficulty in breathing
auriscope ['ɔ:rɪskəʊp] (13) instrument for examining the ear
autoclave ['ɔ:təkleɪv] (7) instrument for high pressure steam sterilization

bactericide [bæk'tɪərɪsaɪd] (7) something which kills bacteria
bacteria [bæk'tɪərɪə] (7) small organisms, some which damage the body
bacteriostatic [ˌbæktɪərɪəʊ'stætɪk] (7) stopping the growth of bacteria
bed-bath ['bed bɑ:θ] (4) a method of bathing a patient in bed
bed-block ['bed blɒk] (10) a piece of material for raising one end of a bed
bed-cradle ['bed ˌkreɪdl] (10) a frame put over the end of the bed to keep blankets off the legs and feet
bedpan ['bedpæn] (4) pot used by bed-ridden patients for excretion
bile [baɪl] (20) a liquid produced by the liver
bilirubin [ˌbɪlɪ'ru:bɪn] product of the breakdown of haemoglobin*
bladder ['blædəʳ] (20) a sac containing urine, see diagram on p.119
blood pressure ['blʌdˌpreʃəʳ] (8) pressure on the walls of the blood vessels
bowels [baʊəlz] (17) intestine, gut; to have one's bowels open (17) to pass faeces
breast [brest] (2) upper front part of the body between the neck and abdomen
bronchiectasis [ˌbrɒŋkɪ'ektəsɪs] (19) widening of the bronchial tubes following infection
bronchus ['brɒŋkəs] (19) one of the two branches into which the windpipe divides
bruise [bru:z] (2) a blue discolouration of the skin due to blood under the skin
buttock ['bʌtək] (2) muscles of the bottom

C° [si:] = **Centigrade** ['sentɪgreɪd] (23) degrees on a centigrade thermometer

calf [kɑ:f] (2) fleshy part of the back of the leg below the knee

carcinoma [ˌkɑ:sɪ'nəʊmə] (19) a malignant growth

cardiac ['kɑ:dɪæk] (4) of the heart

catheter ['kæθɪtəʳ] (4) tube to take out urine

C.S.S.D. [si: es es 'di:] (5) Central Sterile Supply Department, department where supplies are sterilized

cerebral ['serəbrəl] (4) of the brain

Cetrimide ['setrɪmaɪd] (5) antiseptic

clammy ['klæmɪ] (18) cold and damp

clinical ['klɪnɪkəl] (4) observation and treatment of patients as opposed to theoretical study of disease

coma ['kəʊmə] (19) complete loss of consciousness

compound *(n)* (fracture*) ['kɒmpaʊnd] (8) where a broken bone breaks the surrounding tissue (skin)

consciousness ['kɒnʃəsnəs] (10) the state of being conscious of one's surroundings

constipation [ˌkɒnstɪ'peɪʃən] (21) difficulty in getting rid of faeces

consultant [kən'sʌltənt] (12) senior doctor in a hospital

contraction [kən'trækʃən] (23) shortening of muscles

contusion [kən'tju:ʃən] (8) a bruise

convalescence [ˌkɒnvə'lesəns] (11) rest after illness

corpuscles ['kɔ:pʌsəls] (18) red and white blood cells in the blood

cross infection [ˌkrɒs in'fekʃən] (12) infection passed from one patient to the other

crutch [krʌtʃ] (10) wood or metal support to help a patient walk

cuticle ['kju:tɪkəl] (18) the dead skin surrounding a nail

cyanosed ['saɪənəʊzd] (18) a bluish colour of the skin

cyst [sɪst] (24) a sac containing liquid

cytological [ˌsaɪtə'lɒdʒɪkəl] (1) study of the cells of the body

defaecation [ˌdi:fə'keɪʃən] (21) passing faeces from the body

dehydrated [ˌdi:haɪ'dreɪtɪd] (18) lack of fluid

dermatology [ˌdɜ:mə'tɒlədʒɪ] (1) the science of the skin

dermis ['dɜ:mɪs] (18) the layer of skin just below the surface

diabetes [daɪə'bi:ti:s] (19) illness caused by the pancreas not working properly

diarrhoea [daɪə'rɪə] (19) liquid faeces

digest *(v)* [daɪ'dʒest] (21) to change food to a substance which can be absorbed by the body

disinfect [ˌdɪsɪn'fekt] (7) to kill germs

dissecting [dɪ'sektɪŋ] (24) cutting in pieces

distension [dɪs'tenʃən] (24) swelling

dose [dəʊs] (4) amount of medicine taken

drainage ['dreɪnɪdʒ] (22) any method of taking liquid away from the body

dressing ['dresɪŋ] (4) medicines and bandages put on a wound

drug [drʌg] (4) chemical substances used to alter the state of mind or body

duct [dʌkt] (18) tube

duodenum [ˌdju:əʊ'di:nəm] (20) first part of the small intestine, see diagram on p. 110

dyspnoea [dɪsp'nɪə] (19) difficult, laboured breathing

dysuria [dɪs'jʊərɪə] (22) difficult, painful urination

elated [ɪ'leɪtɪd] (17) unusually, extremely happy

emesis ['emɪsɪs] (20) vomiting

E.N.T. [i: en ti:] (1) ear, nose and throat

epidermis [ˌepɪ'dɜ:mɪs] (18) outside layer of skin

excise *(v)* [ek'saɪz] (9) to cut out

excreta [ek'skri:tə] (7) waste matter (faeces, urine)

expectorate (v) [eks'pektəreɪt] (19) to spit

expiration [ˌekspɪ'reɪʃən] (23) a breath blown out

F° [ef] = **Fahrenheit** ['færənhaɪt] (23) a temperature scale

faeces [ˈfiːsiːz] (7) solid waste matter of the body

fever [ˈfiːvə^{r}] (18) when the body temperature is above normal

fibula [ˈfɪbjʊlə] (8) long thin bone on outside of lower leg

flatus [ˈfleɪtəs] (20) gas in the stomach or intestines

flush [flʌʃ] (12) to go red

forceps [ˈfɔːseps] (5) two-pronged instrument, see p. 27

foreign body [ˌfɒrən ˈbɒdɪ] (19) something inside the body that should not be there, e.g. germ, etc.

fracture [ˈfræktʃə^{r}] (8) a break in a bone

gag [gæg] (10) instrument to keep the mouth open, see p. 61

gall [gɔːl] (20) see bile

gallipot [ˈgælɪpɒt] (5) small vessel for lotions, see p. 28

gauze [gɔːz] (5) an open woven cloth used for dressing wounds

genitals [ˈdʒenɪtlz] (2) sexual organs

Gentian violet [ˌdʒenʃən ˈvaɪələt] (7) —a purple coloured antiseptic

geriatrics [ˌdʒerɪˈætrɪks] (1) medical care of old people

gland [glænd] (18) an organ or structure which produces a secretion

grab rail [ˈgræb reɪl] (12) a hand rail to steady patients who have difficulty in walking

graze [greɪz] (2) to scratch

groin [grɔɪn] (2) the area between the belly and thighs

gynaecology [ˌgaɪnəˈkɒlədʒɪ] (1) study of women's diseases

haematology [ˌhiːməˈtɒlədʒɪ] (1) study of the blood

haematuria [ˌhiːməˈtjʊərɪə] (22) blood in the urine

haemoglobin [ˌhiːməˈgləʊbɪn] red part of the blood which combines with and releases oxygen

haemoptysis [hiːmɒptəsɪs] (19) coughing up blood

haemorrhage [ˈhemərɪdʒ] (4) bleeding

Hibitane [ˈhɪbɪteɪn] (5) Chlorhexidine [klɔːˈheksɪdiːn], an antiseptic

histology [hɪsˈtɒlədʒɪ] (1) study of the tissues of the body

history [ˈhɪstərɪ] (8) patient's previous medical record

houseman [ˈhaʊsm n] (10) junior hospital doctor

hyperpnoea [ˌhaɪpəpˈnɪə] (19) deep breathing

hyperpyrexia [ˌhaɪpəpaɪˈreksɪə] (18) feverish

hypothalamus [ˌhaɪpəʊˈθæləməs] (23) below the thalamus (collection of grey matter in the uppermost part of the brain)

immerse [ɪˈmɜːs] (5) to put below the surface of a liquid or gas

immunize [ˈɪmjʊnaɪz] (8) to make safe against a disease usually by injection of dead germ of the disease

incontinence [inˈkɒntɪnəns] (22) unable to control the emptying of the bladder or bowels

indigestible [ˌɪndaɪˈdʒestəbəl] (21) difficult to digest

infant [ˈɪnfənt] (24) a baby less than a year old

infarction [ɪnˈfɑːkʃən] (4) death of a piece of tissue because the blood supply has stopped

infection [ɪnˈfekʃən] (8) the invasion of the body by a germ

inflammation [ˌɪnfləˈmeɪʃən] the reaction of living tissue to injury

infusion [ɪnˈfjuːʒən] (4) fluid put into the body

injection [ɪnˈdʒekʃən] (4) the act of putting a fluid into the body's tissues

intensive care unit [ɪnˌtensɪv ˈkeə juːnɪt] (1) unit where seriously ill patients receive intensive treatment

intercostal [ˌɪntəˈkɒstəl] (24) between the ribs

intestine [ɪnˈtestɪn] (20) the bowels

intramuscular [ˌintrəˈmʌskjʊlə^{r}] (10) within a muscle

intravenous (**I.V.**) [ˌɪntrəˈviːnəs] (4) (22) within or into a vein

Iodine ['aɪədi:n] (7) antiseptic used for cleaning wounds

irrigate ['ɪrɪgəɪt] (7) to pour liquid in, e.g. *to irrigate the eye* to wash out a foreign body

irritant ['ɪrɪtənt] (19) something causing an itch

jaundice ['dʒɔ:ndɪs] (18) raised bilirubin which may cause* in the blood cause yellowing of the skin

kidney ['kɪdnɪ] (5) (22) two glands which secrete urine

kidney dish ['kɪdnɪ dɪʃ] (5) dish, so called because of its shape. see p. 30

lacerate ['læsəreɪt] (8) to cut

larynx ['lærɪŋks] (19) the organ of voice

laxative ['læksətɪv] (21) a mild drug to open the bowels

lay up [ˌleɪ 'ʌp] (13) to arrange (usually instruments)

linen ['lɪnɪn] (7) sheets and pillowcases

liver ['lɪvəʳ] (20) a gland which plays an important part in breaking down protein

lobe [ləʊb] (19) rounded section

long stay [ˌlɒŋ 'steɪ] (1) a patient who will be in hospital for a long time

lotion ['ləʊʃən] (5) liquid medicine applied to the skin

lung [lʌŋ] (19) organs of breathing

Lysol ['laɪsɒl] (5) a disinfectant

malignant [ˌmə'lɪgnənt] likely to be incurable

medical social worker [ˌmedɪkəl 'səʊʃəl ˌwɜ:kəʳ] (14) worker who helps patients with problems outside the hospital

melaena [mə'li:nə] (21) black tarry faeces

membrane ['membreɪn] a thin lining or covering

metabolic [metə'bɒlɪk] (22) about metabolism [me'tæbəlɪzm] the processes of chemical change in the body

micro-organism ['maɪkrəʊ 'ɔ:gənɪsəm] (7) a cell which can only be seen under a microscope; bacteria, virus, etc.

micturition [ˌmɪktʃʊə'rɪʃən] (22) urination

morphine ['mɔ:fi:n] (8) a powerful pain-killing drug

mucoid ['mju:kɔɪd] (18) like mucus

mucopurulent [ˌmju:kəʊ'pjʊərʊlənt] (19) pus in the mucus

mucus ['mju:kəs] (19) slimy substance lubricating the respiratory, alimentary surfaces, etc.

nasal ['neɪzəl] (19) concerning the nose

nausea ['nɔ:sɪə] (10) feeling of sickness

navel ['neɪvəl] (2) umbilicus, depression in the stomach muscle wall

nipple ['nɪpəl] (2) hard lump on surface of each breast

Nobecutane ['nəʊbəˌkju:teɪn] (5) artificial skin sprayed on a wound

no touch [ˌnəʊ 'tʌtʃ] (9) aseptic procedure where nothing that has not been sterilized touches the patient

obstetrics [ɒb'stetrɪks] (1) medical care in pregnancy and child birth

occupational therapy [ˌɒkjupeɪʃənəl 'θerəpɪ] (1) use of occupations (basket-making, etc) to help mental or physical disorders

odour ['əʊdəʳ] (21) smell

oesophagus [i:'sɒfəgəs] (20) the gullet, tube from the pharynx to the stomach

oliguria [ˌɒlɪ'gjʊərɪə] (22) insufficient secretion of urine

optimal ['ɒptɪməl] (13) best possible

oral ['ɔ:rəl] (19) by mouth

organic [ɔ:'gænɪk] (21) concerning an organ

orthopaedics [ˌɔ:θə'pi:dɪks] (1) surgery of the locomotor system (bones)

orthopnoea [ˌɔ:θəp'nɪə] (19) breathlessness requiring an upright sitting position

out-patient ['aʊtpeɪʃənt] (1) patient who is not treated in hospital

paediatrics [ˌpi:dɪ'ætrɪks] (1) medical care of children

pallid ['pælɪd] (18) white (pale) skin colouring

pancreas ['pæŋkrɪəs] (20) an organ which secretes pancreatic juice, see p. 110

pass urine [ˌpɑːs 'jʊərɪn] (17 to urinate, pass water

pathology [pə'θɒlədʒɪ] (1) study of cause and nature of disease

penicillin [ˌpenɪ'sɪlɪn] (11) the first antibiotic discovered

Pethidine ['peθɪdɪn] (10) strong pain-killing drug

pharynx ['færɪŋks] (19) the hollow at the back of the mouth opening onto the oesophagus

Phenol ['fiːnɒl] (7) disinfectant

phlegm [flem] (19) mucus from the bronchus

physician [fɪ'zɪʃən] (1) doctor of medicine rather than surgery

physiology [ˌfɪzɪ'ɒlədʒɪ] (3) study of the normal functions of the body

physiotherapy [ˌfɪzɪəʊ'θerəpɪ] (1) controlled exercises

pigment ['pɪgmənt] (21) colouring matter in the body

pleura ['plʊərə] (19) membrane* covering the surface of the lung

pneumonia [njuː'məʊnɪə] (4) inflammation of the lung

polyuria [ˌpɒlɪ'jʊərɪə] (22) large amount of urine

pore [pɔː^r] (18) a minute opening in the skin

posterior [pɒ'stɪərɪə^r] (2) at the back

post- (operative, natal, etc.) [pəʊst] after

pre- [priː] before

premedication [ˌpriːmedɪ'keɪʃən] (8) drug given before the administration of general anaesthetic

probe [prəʊb] (5) an instrument for investigating the depth and direction of a wound, see p. 29

proctoscope ['prɒktəskəʊp] (13) an instrument for examining the rectum

Proflavine [prəʊ'fleɪviːn] (7) an antiseptic

proteinuria [ˌprəʊtiːn'jʊərɪə] (22) protein in the urine

psychiatry [saɪ'kaɪətrɪ] (1) science of diagnosis and treatment of mental illness

psychology [saɪ'kɒlədʒɪ] (1) study of human behaviour

pulmonary ['pʌlmənərɪ] (19) concerned with the lungs

pulse [pʌls] (8) regular beat of the arteries as blood is pumped round them by the heart

purulent ['pjuːrjuːlənt] (19) pusy

pus [pʌs] (7) yellowish (usually) coloured liquid formed in certain infections

putty ['pʌtɪ] (21) pale grey

pyrexia [paɪ'reksɪə] (18) raised temperature

queasy ['kwiːzɪ] (20) sick feeling

radial ['reɪdɪəl] (24) the outside

radiology [ˌreɪdɪ'ɒlədʒɪ] (1) diagnosis of disease by the use of x-rays

rash [ræʃ] (2) skin eruption

raw [rɔː] (9) when the skin is partly removed from the body's surface

reaction [rɪ'ækʃən] (22) response to a stimulus

receiver [rɪ'siːvə^r] (5) dish, see p.30

rectum ['rektəm] (20) lower part of the large intestine

reduce [rɪ'djuːs] (9) realign two parts of a broken bone

reflex ['riːfleks] (19) an involuntary movement of tissue

respiration [ˌrespɪ'reɪʃən] (9) breathing

rib [rɪb] (24) bone of the chest

ribbon gauze [ˌrɪbən 'gɔːz] (5) gauze about 1.5 cm. wide used for packing wounds

salivary ['sælɪvərɪ] (20) concerning saliva, spittle

sanitary ['sænɪtrɪ] (7) concerned with the preservation of health

scalpel ['skælpəl] (6) surgical knife

scaly ['skeɪlɪ] (18) flakes of skin

scar [skɑː^r] (2) mark of a healed wound

secretion [sɪ'kriːʃən] (8) a substance formed by or concentrated in a gland

semi- [ˌsemɪ-] (21) partly

shock [ʃɒk] (8) disturbance of circulation of the blood produced by severe illness or injury

side effect ['saɪd ɪˌfekt] (4) an unwanted change produced by giving a drug
sinus ['saɪnəs] (5) a hollow, cavity
sluice [slu:s] (11) explained on p. 79
soiled ['sɔɪld] (5) dirty
sore [sɔ:ʳ] (2) *(n)* an irritation on the skin *(adv)* painful.
specific gravity [spəˌsɪfɪk 'grævɪtɪ] (22) the weight of a substance compared with an equal volume of water
speculum ['spekjʊləm] (13) an instrument used to hold the walls of a cavity apart so that its interior can be examined, see p. 80
sphygmomanometer [ˌsfɪgməʊmə'nɒmɪtəʳ] (10) an instrument used for measuring blood pressure, see p. 60
sprain [spreɪn] (2) injury to the soft tissue surrounding a joint
sputum ['spju:təm] (7) matter coughed up from the respiratory organs
S.R.N. [ˌes ɑ:r 'en] (1) State Registered Nurse
sterilize ['sterəlaɪz] (5) to make free of bacteria, to make incapable of reproduction
sternum ['stɜ:nəm] (24) the flat bone in the front of the chest
stertorous ['stɜ:tərəs] (19) breathing like snoring
stethoscope ['steθəskəʊp] (9) instrument for listening to sounds inside the body
stool [stu:l] (21) faeces
stretcher ['stretʃəʳ] (8) length of canvas between two poles for carrying patients
subcutaneous [ˌsʌbkju:'teɪnɪəs] (18) beneath the skin
Sudol [su:dol] (5) a disinfectant
superficial [ˌsu:pə'fɪʃəl] (23) concerning the surface
sustain [sə'steɪn] (8) to suffer an injury
suture ['su:tʃəʳ] (9) stitch
swab [swɒb] (5) (7) a small piece of cotton wool or gauze used for soaking up liquid
symptom ['sɪmptəm] (19) sign of illness
syringe [sɪ'rɪndʒ] (6) piston-fitted cylinder into which liquid is sucked and then injected
tactile ['tæktaɪl] (18) concerning the sense of touch
tarry ['tɑ:rɪ] (21) *(adj)* black and sticky
tetanus ['tetənəs] (8) lockjaw, disease marked by spasms of the voluntary muscles
thermometer [θə'mɒmɪtəʳ] (4) instrument for measuring the temperature of the body
thoracic [θɔ:'ræsɪk] (24) concerning the chest cavity
thrombosis [θrɒm'bəʊsɪs] (4) a blood clot
tibia ['tɪbɪə] (8) the shin bone
tincture ['tɪŋktʃəʳ] (7) solution of a drug in alcohol
tissue ['tiʃju:] (7) collection of cells or fibres of similar function, forming a structure
tonsils ['tɒnsəlz] (14) small bodies embedded in the fauces between the palatine arch in the throat
toxic ['tɒksɪk] (7) poisonous
t.p.r. [ˌti: pi: 'ɑ:ʳ] (4) temperature, pulse and respiration
trachea [trə'kɪə] (19) windpipe
trolley ['trɒlɪ] (4) wheeled vehicle for carrying goods
tuberculosis [tju:ˌbɜ:kjʊ'ləʊsɪs] (19) disease caused by tubercle bacillus

unconscious [ʌn'kɒnʃəs] (9) state of being insensible
undigested [ˌʌndaɪ'dʒestɪd] (21) not digested
unsterile [ʌn'steraɪl] (5) not sterile
uraemia [jʊə'ri:mɪə] (19) condition due to failure of the kidneys
urea [jʊə'rɪə] (22) the waste product from protein
ureter [jʊə'ri:təʳ] (22) tube passing from each kidney to the bladder
urethra [jʊə'ri:θrə] (22) tube from the bladder through which urine is excreted
urinal ['jʊərɪnəl] (4) pot or fixture for passing urine
urine ['jʊərɪn] (7) liquid waste matter

excreted from the kidneys
urinometer [ˌjʊərɪˈnɒmətəʳ] (13) instrument for measuring the specific gravity of urine

vaginal [vəˈdʒaɪnəl] (13) concerning the vagina, the passage from the cervix to the vulva
venerology [ˌvenəˈrɒlədʒɪ] (1) study of diseases caused by sexual intercourse
ventricle [ˈventrɪkəl] (24) a cavity, here the lower chamber in the heart
vomit [ˈvɒmɪt] (20) to bring up vomitus
vomitus [ˈvɒmɪtəs] (20) outflow of the contents of the stomach through the mouth
vulva [vʌlvə] external female sex organ

x-ray [ˈeks reɪ] (1) short rays of the electromagnetic spectrum for photographing structures within the body